40 Days to Enlightened Eating

Journey to Optimal Weight, Health, Energy, and Vitality

Elise Cantrell

BALBOA.
PRESS
A DIVISION OF HAY HOUSE

Library of Congress Control Number: 2012912353

Balboa Press books may be ordered through booksellers or by contacting:

Balboa Press
A Division of Hay House
1663 Liberty Drive
Bloomington, IN 47403
www.balboapress.com
1-(877) 407-4847

ISBN: 978-1-4525-5467-9 (sc)
ISBN: 978-1-4525-5469-3 (hc)
ISBN: 978-1-4525-5468-6 (e)

Because of the dynamic nature of the Internet, any web addresses or links contained in this book may have changed since publication and may no longer be valid. The views expressed in this work are solely those of the author and do not necessarily reflect the views of the publisher, and the publisher hereby disclaims any responsibility for them.

The author of this book does not dispense medical advice or prescribe the use of any technique as a form of treatment for physical, emotional, or medical problems without the advice of a physician, either directly or indirectly. The intent of the author is only to offer information of a general nature to help you in your quest for emotional and spiritual well-being. In the event you use any of the information in this book for yourself, which is your constitutional right, the author and the publisher assume no responsibility for your actions.

Any people depicted in stock imagery provided by Thinkstock are models, and such images are being used for illustrative purposes only.
Certain stock imagery © Thinkstock.

Printed in the United States of America

Balboa Press rev. date: 10/09/2012

Contents

Preface: How My Own Journey Began

In my early 20's I was a high school teacher. I taught in an overcrowded school in South Carolina, with 35 students in each class. The school was a poor rural school, and many of the students came to me with very different values and a very different way of life than I had grown up with. Violence could break out at a moment's notice! The students came to me with very serious personal problems that I was not trained or equipped as a 23 year old art teacher, to help them face. I came home every day very stressed and depleted! One day I came across a magazine article about Yoga, and it explained and depicted five or six Yoga poses. I tore out the article and came home every day from teaching and practiced the poses. I got to where I could hold them longer and longer. I noticed I felt better, less stressed, stronger, firmer and more relaxed. I finally went and bought my first Yoga book, called <u>Sivananda Yoga</u>. Page by page, I taught myself the poses. Once I became pregnant with my first child, I let Yoga fall by the wayside . . .

However, it was not long after becoming a young mom, when I got a severe case of food poisoning at an upscale Italian restaurant. This illness evolved into a severe case of irritable bowel syndrome (IBS). With the IBS, I was in terrible pain from morning to night with intestinal cramping. While my toddler napped, I curled up into a ball, praying she would sleep so I could just deal with the pain. When I ate the pain would worsen, and anything I ate would immediately be expelled from my body through diarrhea or vomiting. It was as if my body had determined that all food was the enemy and it rejected everything I put in my mouth! I could not keep food in long enough to digest or absorb it, and I became painfully thin. As I helplessly grew thinner and thinner, I became emaciated and it was terrifying to have no control over something as basic as eating and digestion. The worst part however, was the pain. I have had two children and experienced labor and childbirth twice. IBS was like being in labor 24 hours a day. I still remember the pain vividly! I could barely function, and was unable to sleep as the sharp cramping plagued me day and night. As sick as I was, the doctors were unable to help. At the time, there was very little that could be done to relieve IBS. Nothing they tried was effective. The doctors essentially gave up on me saying, "No one has ever died from IBS!"

After months of weakness, pain and frustration with conventional medicine's inability to help, I turned to alternative medicine, specifically Yoga, Ayurveda and hypnosis. I began to practice Yoga again and noticed it helped tremendously with the pain and cramping, and it helped ease the tension and stress that go along with illness and pain. It also allowed me to relax enough to get healing rest and sleep. Inspired by the results which accompanied Yoga, I began to read books on Ayurvedic healing. With determination, I adhered to the recommendations for healing IBS, and for the first time I began to improve! I was astounded that something so ancient could help me when modern medicine was incapable! I also underwent hypnosis with a licensed hypnotherapist who just happened to be my own dad! I felt empowered by taking charge of my own body and my own health, and within a year, I completely recovered. For some people, IBS is a crippling life-long illness. For me, this was the start of my journey into Yoga and Ayurveda, health and healing. It is from this place, where my passion for these ancient healing sciences has blossomed.

After healing completely, I went back to my old ways of eating, and became sporadic with my practice of Yoga. A year or so later I became pregnant. During my pregnancy I gained nearly 40 pounds. Convinced that it would again drop off quickly after the baby was born, I was devastated when that didn't happen. I tried every diet and extreme exercise regime du jour, but the weight did not budge! Finally, I turned back to that which had helped me in the past, Yoga and Ayurveda. Once again it worked! I now weigh what I weighed in high school, and I feel the best I have felt in my life. I have become so passionate about the Vedic healing sciences of Yoga and Ayurveda, that I became a certified Yoga instructor and Ayurvedic Lifestyle Counselor. I began to teach workshops to help others find their optimal weight, health, energy and vitality. This became quite popular and word quickly began to spread. A book began to unfold from these workshops, and incredibly the book seemed to write itself! It is my honor and pleasure to share with you the fruit of these experiences, <u>40 Days to Enlightened Eating.</u>

40 Days to Enlightened Eating:

A Journey to Optimal Weight, Health, Energy and Vitality

By Elise Cantrell

Introduction

"Our Physical body is a representation of our past and not our future."
~Laura Toolin

I would like to invite you on a journey. The destination is your ideal self. On this journey, you will be led along a path which has gone untraveled by most of us in the western world. Along this path are many ancient secrets. These secrets are the avenue to a better self, better health and a better life. These secrets involve what and how we are designed to eat. Long ago these were not secrets, but common practice. Today this wisdom has long been lost. Harnessing the time-tested wisdom of the ancient Vedic sciences of Yoga and Ayurveda, you will rediscover eating and food. Along this path you will discover how to eat the way we were originally intended, according to our design. By discovering this secret alone, the body, mind and spirit can be transformed in just 40 days. In 40 days you will uncover the optimal you!

For the next 40 days, there will be no counting calories, fat, carbs or points. There are no expensive bars, supplements, pre-prepared meals, or shakes. There is no eating only grapefruit or cabbage soup. This new way of eating did not originate in Beverly Hills or South Beach, but from long ago and far away. This book is not about becoming super-model thin, but about finding your optimal, healthy weight and metabolism. These 40 days aren't only about losing weight, but about gaining health, energy and vitality. Many eating plans cause weight-loss at the expense of energy and health. This plan is different. This plan is developed to lighten not only your body, but the mind and spirit as well. For the next 40 days, each day is a chapter in the book. Each day and chapter will layer on a new aspect of eating and food as it relates to the body, mind and spirit. Each day is one step closer to transformation.

In our search to look younger, feel more energetic, and become slimmer and healthier, westerners have tried every new "fad" diet and weight loss scheme "du jour". And the results . . . we are fatter and less healthy than ever before in history! Fads clearly don't work. There is no better time than now to rediscover ancient, time tested solutions to weight, health, energy and vitality. The 5000 year old sciences of Yoga and Ayurveda contain ancient wisdom and knowledge that is more practical now than ever, and more needed now than ever, here in the modern era.

What is Ayurveda?

Ayurveda is an ancient healing science from India. Ayurveda is the medical or healing sister science of Yoga. Ayurveda literally means the "science of life". This 5000 year old practice of health and healing aims at bringing the body, mind and spirit back into harmony with each other and with nature. Acknowledging that human beings themselves are a part of nature, Ayurveda teaches that when the human being is in balance with the rhythms of nature, the result is health and vitality. Ayurveda focuses on maintaining and restoring a person's natural state of balance and harmony mentally, physically, spiritually and emotionally. Ayurveda employs a variety of methods including diet, lifestyle adjustments, detoxification practices, meditation techniques, herbs, Yoga postures, and breathing excercises, prescribed for specific ailments to shift momentum towards health and healing.

Ayurveda recognizes that each human being has a unique individual make-up or constitution. It guides the individual to make the right choices for their unique disposition in order to maintain balance for optimal health. A fundamental Ayurvedic philosophy is that "food is medicine, and medicine is food." An Ayurvedic proverb is *"When diet is wrong, medicine is of no use; when diet is correct, medicine is of no need."* Ayurveda sees natural whole foods as the concentrated intelligent energy or life-force of the universe. These foods have the innate power within them to heal and transform.

What is Yoga?

Yoga comes from the root word *yuj* meaning to join, yoke or unite the body, breath, mind and spirit. This practice was developed by ancient sages who passed it on for centuries from teacher to student. It was developed as a system of physical exercises for maintaining wellness, and as a system of holistic health and healing. Yoga was intended to bring healing and well-being through physical movements which were designed to regulate energy flow through the body. Energy blockages are thought to be the sites where disease accumulates. Unless blockages are removed, eventually disease begins to manifest with physical symptoms. Areas of stiffness, tension or tightness such as stiff joints and muscles are often areas where energy flow is restricted or blocked. Yoga helps release tension, move stuck energy, and activate the body's innate healing power. By maintaining and restoring proper energy flow, Yoga is said to return the mind, body and spirit to a natural state of health and balance. The physical practice of Yoga, is helpful in healing and in maintaining wellness. Specific Yoga poses were once given as a "prescription" for healing a given ailment. Regular Yoga practice is said to maintain proper energy flow throughout the body and stimulate immune function promoting ongoing health.

The science of Yoga is a system whose exact origins have been lost in antiquity. Archeology has unearthed artifacts depicting figures in "lotus pose" dating back 5000 years. Yoga appears to have spread through India and Tibet and was practiced by Hindus and Buddhists alike. Yoga has continued to evolve and adapt to the different needs of varying cultures, creeds and populations, over the centuries to the present. Yoga appears to be timeless. Yoga is not a religion in and of itself, however it does emphasize the importance of having a spiritual practice and a personal relationship with God. Yoga teaches that whatever your faith tradition may be, you should follow it wholeheartedly. The Yoga system endorses a set of ethical principles to strive towards including truthfulness, non-harming, and non-greed. Yoga also emphasizes meditation as the mental aspect of the practice. Yoga is unique in that it holds the individual responsible for the health and well-being of their own mind, body and spirit.

What does your "ideal" self look like?

Take a moment to visualize your ideal self. What is your appearance like? How do you feel? What is your overall mood or emotional tone? What is your energy level? Envision your hair, nails, skin, health and weight. How youthful do you look and feel? How do you move through life? How is your life right now different from your ideal? How peaceful and harmonious is your spirit? Today is the beginning of your journey towards that ideal self. That "you" is standing there waiting at the end of the 40 days. It is my honor to guide you along the path to the optimal you. I will be with you every day leading you forward. Each day is a step towards enlightened eating.

Why 40 Days?

What is so special about 40 days? First of all, it takes 21 days for new habits to create new neuro-pathways in the brain, but 40 days is optimal time necessary for those new neuro-pathways to become fixed and lasting. 40 days is an ideal length of time for the neuro-pathways of old habits to weaken and fade, and let the new ones take over permanently. It is said that "motivation is what gets you started, but it is habit which keeps you going."

40 days also has a powerful spiritual significance across many ideologies, particularly Judaism, Christianity and Islam. 40-day time periods are mentioned in the Bible 22 times. Moses fasted 40 days before he received "enlightenment" in the form of the Ten Commandments. Jesus spent 40 days praying and fasting in the wilderness after his baptism. It rained 40 days and 40 nights during the great Biblical flood . . . a great cleansing of the Earth, if you will. Many Christians observe Lent, a 40-day time of fasting in preparation for Easter. In the Islamic religion, Ramadan lasts 40 days. It too is a time of fasting and reconnection to spirit. In the Kabbalah tradition, a form of ancient Jewish mysticism, 40 days is the period of time it takes to establish new patterns, and make them lasting parts of our lives. Each of these 40 day time periods is about transformation. Over the next 40 days you too will undergo transformation in the body as well as the mind and spirit. 40 days is the ideal amount of time to reset the appetite, cravings, taste buds, and rejuvenate the whole self. In 40 days you can gently and fully detoxify the bodily systems with noticeable results.

It is important to note that during the next 40 days you are going to face temptation. During his 40 days in the desert, Jesus faced temptation three times. The Buddha faced temptation three times before he was enlightened. Like Jesus and Buddha, the incarnated Hindu deity, Krishna was tempted three times in the wilderness, and the Islamic prophet Mohammed was allegedly tempted. Temptation is part of the change process. Keep in mind that it is during the times when you struggle with temptation and prevail; these are sacred moments which spark transformation. Know that it does take effort to change habits that are deeply rooted, but also know that with effort, grace and faith, it can be done. I have seen many people following this plan transform before my eyes, and you can too.

How to use this book:

Over the next 40 days, take one day at a time. Do not read ahead to the next day. Just as in life, it is important to be fully present to the day at hand and not be always looking ahead. Each day of the next 40 days will add a new layer and new insight into what it means to eat in an enlightened way. In order to "digest" and integrate this new way of eating, it is important to proceed one day at a time.

Each day's chapter will explain new concepts, and then suggest how to integrate them in "Focus for Today." There is a daily "Journal" suggestion to help personalize the teachings and practices. "Recipes" and a "Daily Food Journal" are also included each day to support your transformation. The appendices provide additional supportive material relevant to many chapters and include a suggested grocery list, an easy guide to the 3-day cleanse, a recipe index, frequently asked questions, students greatest insights over the 40 days, ways to save money while eating healthy, and healthy food resources.

In 40 days, you will see your body transform, as your optimal physical blueprint emerges. Unnatural deposits of fat will disappear as your metabolism awakens and is no longer weighted down by toxins. Your skin, hair and nails will become healthy, luminous and youthful as they reflect the newfound nourishment the body is receiving. You will feel a dramatic improvement in your energy, stamina, and vitality. Your mind will sharpen and focus. You will notice a sense of emotional balance and improved mood. Perhaps most surprisingly, you will notice your spiritual connection deepen as your spirit is no longer dulled by heavy or unnatural foods. During the next 40 days, each day will bring you one step closer to new healthy patterns of eating which will be transforming to the body, mind and spirit! You will be pressing your own "reset" button over the next 40 days, with changes which will last a lifetime!

"There are two mistakes one can make along the path to the truth: never starting, and not going all the way." ~the Buddha

Day 1: Beginner's Mind

"In order for us to learn something new, often we first have to unlearn."
~Elise Cantrell

Suzuki Roshi wisely summarizes the concept of beginner's mind in his statement: *"In the beginner's mind, there are many possibilities, in the expert's mind, there are few."* Very often we let our "knowing" get in the way of our learning. Our minds are closed by our own preconceptions, judgments, and prejudices. By allowing ourselves to experience "beginner's mind" we suddenly become open to new possibilities and new ways of looking at things. When we become a beginner, we are open for transformation to take place. We create space for grace to flow in.

Today is the start of the journey. Beginning today we will approach eating with "beginner's mind". We will come to eating with a new sense of curiosity. Today we will start over. Starting today, we will approach a new way of eating, full of wonder, investigating and observing what happens when we incorporate new dietary principles. Think of the next 40 days as an experiment. Be willing to embark on a new beginning, try new ideas, set new patterns, and create new habits. Approach the next 40 days with **openness.** With the curiosity of a child, try new foods, different vegetables and fruits, new recipes, and creative cuisine. If you don't cook, try it! Cooking can be fun and creative. The next 40 days is a chance for you to make a new start. It's a chance to reset your taste buds, cravings and appetite. For *"If not now, when?"*~Eckhart Tolle

As adults, we fall into set patterns and react out of routine or anticipation. However, life itself gives us opportunities to embrace beginner's mind. When we ourselves were children, we looked at everything with a sense of wonder and amazement. Children observe things just as they are, without expectations. Again as parents we rediscover the world through our children's eyes, recognizing the amazement inherent in discovering things for the first time. Each January 1, many of us begin again with new zest, a new perspective and a clean slate. Give yourself permission to be a beginner when it comes to eating and food. Clear your mind of preconceptions, old habits, and old ways of doing things and give yourself the gift of starting over with a "beginner's mind". This is what I'm asking you to do with **eating** for the next 40 days. If you can commit to trying a new way of eating for 40 days, I can guarantee transformation!

Beginning today, observe yourself when it comes to eating and food as if you are new to it. Notice what and how much you are eating and drinking, and how often. Begin to read the ingredients of the foods you eat. Closely observe how foods taste and how you feel after eating them. Is the food you are eating something you are actually craving? Is there any anxiety for you around eating and food? Do you feel energized after eating, or heavy and sluggish? How much water are you drinking? How much alcohol? For Day 1, the assignment is to just observe through new eyes how you come to eating and food. This will bring about awareness. Awareness is the important first step towards making change. New awareness will emerge as you embrace beginners mind.

Excerpt from Tao Te Ching 27-Lao Tzu

(interpreted by Steven Mitchell)

A good traveler has no fixed plans,
And is not intent upon arriving.
A good artist lets his intuition
Lead him wherever it wants.
A good scientist has freed himself of concepts
And keeps his mind open to what is.

Focus for Today: Begin these 40 days with openness. Begin as if you are learning to eat for the first time. I suggest going to the grocery store (without kids) and really take time to examine products, read labels and notice new foods. See the grocery store through new eyes. Observe your own eating through new eyes, observe your patterns, habits, preconceptions, and hang-ups. As of today, resolve to come to eating as a complete beginner. Try one new "healthy" food today that you have never before tried, and give it a chance. Cook or prepare something new, or even approach cooking as a new adventure if it is something you never enjoyed before. Open your mind to new things over the next 40 days!

Journal: Am I open to trying new things in life? What gets in my way of trying something new? What do I notice when I try new things? Note any temptations. Are you already tempted to "bolt" from the 40 day plan? How do you respond to these temptations, doubts and fears that are arising?

Notice your skin, hair, nails, your body, and the fit of your clothing as if you were meeting yourself for the first time. Record your observations in your journal. Weigh yourself and jot it down. If you have means to check your body fat percentage, then record it. Measure your waist, hips, upper arms, chest and thighs. These are areas where change will be most noticeable! Note your current state of energy and stamina in your journal as well. Note your mood and emotional tone. Note if you have a lot of ups and downs or mood swings. Also note your spiritual connection, your personal connection to God or spirit. These observations will be the baseline for your journey ahead.

Baseline Observations

You may wish to take a before and after the 40 days photo to motivate you along!

My skin is:

My hair is:

My nails are:

The fit of my clothes is:

I currently wear size:

Areas of my body I'd like to see change: (Describe what you'd like to see change.)

Body fat %:

Waist measurement: (Place measuring tape right at navel.)

Upper hip: (Measure area right over the top part of the pelvis bone.)

Lower hip: (Measure the widest area of the hip, around the hip crease in which the thighs and hip meet.)

Thighs: (Measure around the mid-thigh halfway between hip and knee.)

Upper arms: (Measure around the halfway point between shoulder and elbow.)

Chest: (Place tape around the widest part of the chest, under arms, position right at nipples.)

Energy level:

Recent mood and emotional tone:

Spiritual connection: (Prayer life, meditation, and sense of connection to the Divine, being as specific as you can.)

Sense of focus and concentration:

Recipe of the Day: Something new . . .

Cilantro-Quinoa-Zucchini Corn Fritters on a Bed of Fresh Greens with a Lemon-Garlic-Cilantro Dressing

(Serves 4-Makes 8 Corn Fritters)

(Use organic ingredients where possible.)

The Fritters:
1 small zucchini unpeeled, grated
1 cup organic cut corn, cooked
2 full green onions, chopped
1/3 red bell pepper, chopped into small cubes
1 stalk celery, chopped finely
Hand-full of fresh cilantro leaves, chopped finely
½ cup whole wheat flour (I use whole wheat pastry flour)
2 large organic eggs, beaten
½ cup quinoa in 1 cup water—cook until all water is evaporated
Sea salt and pepper to taste
5 Tbsp extra virgin olive oil

Sautee the bell pepper, celery and zucchini in 1 Tbsp olive oil, just until soft. Remove from heat. Add in cooked quinoa, green onions, flour, eggs, cilantro, salt and pepper. Mix together thoroughly. Form into eight fritters. Place 4 Tbsp olive oil in skillet and add fritters. Cook until both sides are golden brown. Serve warm over bed of greens. Drizzle with dressing recipe below.

Dressing:
2 large cloves garlic
Hand-full fresh cilantro leaves
Juice of 1 small lemon
½ tsp Dijon mustard
2 Tbsp Extra virgin olive oil
½ cup plain Greek yogurt
Blend ingredients thoroughly in blender or food processor.

Daily Food Journal

Date:_____ Intention for the day:_____ Weight:_____

Water: X off one water for every 8 oz. of water that you drink. This includes lemon waters. During a cleanse you should have at least 3 lemon waters daily.

YOGI PLATE ➡

¼ Protein
¼ Whole Grains
½ Veggies

Rate your hunger, mood, energy and after meal satisfaction

1=Low   2=Average   3=High

Time	Meal/Snack	Food/Beverage	Hungry?	Mood?	Energy?	Satisfied?
	Breakfast					
	Snack					
	Lunch					
	Snack					
	Dinner					
	Snack					

At the end of the day, reflect on how many servings you had of the following foods/beverages:

Vegetables (Unlimited)	
Whole Grains (Women 1 -3)	
Fruit (Aim for 2)	
Protein (Aim for 3 or more)	

Did I Avoid?	Yes	No	How Much?
Alcohol			
Soft Drinks			
White Sugar			
Artificial Sweeteners			
Processed Food			
Fast Food			

Alert! Use Meat Sparingly

Consume meat no more than 3 times a week!

List your observations and insights for the day. These include successes and behaviors that need attention:
_____
_____
_____
_____
_____

Day 2: A Clean Slate—Putting Beginner's Mind into Action

"A journey of a thousand miles begins with a single step."
~Lao Tzu

One way to create a new beginning is start things off with a "clean slate", by detoxifying and "resetting" the body. In Ayurveda, it is considered essential to periodically cleanse the body of accumulated toxins. Just as we "spring clean" our homes, so too we should cleanse the body, our spirit's temporary home. In Ayurveda, toxic build-up in the body is referred to as *ama*. *Ama* or toxins build up in the body due to exposure to pollutants, pesticides, chemicals, processed food, artificial colors, flavors, additives and preservatives. *Ama* can also accumulate in the body due to stress, poor sleep quality, heavy foods, a diet heavy in meat, consuming excess alcohol, as well as having poor digestion. The older we get, the body's natural ability to rid itself of toxins or *ama* becomes progressively less and less efficient. This causes us to age faster and faster and our metabolism to slow as the years go by. It is said that physical aging accelerates every 7 years. Periodically incorporating a cleansing regime can help to renew youthfulness and vitality, slow the hands of time and reinvigorate the metabolism. Maintaining a diet and lifestyle which reduce the accumulation of *ama* helps slow the acceleration of aging, while preventing the metabolism from slowing. Today we are going to press our own internal "reset" button by beginning a 3-day cleanse. Take the quiz below to determine whether you have accumulated toxins in your system weighing down your metabolism, immune system and overall energy.

Self-Quiz: 18 Signs You Have Accumulated *Ama* (Toxins)

1. Does your tongue have a brown, yellow or thick white coating when you wake up in the morning?
2. Does your breath have a sharp smell?
3. Do you frequently find yourself drowsy after a meal?
4. Do you feel fatigued, sluggish or lethargic during the day, even after a good night's sleep?
5. Do you crave junk food, alcohol, caffeine or sweets?
6. Are you lacking motivation or enthusiasm for life, often just "going through the motions"?
7. Does your mind seem hazy or "spaced out"?
8. Have you noticed bloating, abdominal discomfort, cramping or intestinal gas after eating?
9. Do you have bouts of constipation or irregular bowel movements?
10. Does your stool sink?
11. Do you experience unexplained aches, pains or joint discomfort?
12. Do you frequently notice phlegm or congestion in the nose, throat or waste?
13. Do you have difficulty sleeping, restless sleep, or waking in the night?
14. Is your energy level inconsistent or low?
15. Is your skin clear and lustrous, or do you notice pimples, acne, or a dull complexion?
16. Are your eyes clear and bright or dull with yellowish or grayish whites?
17. Is your urine cloudy?
18. Does your perspiration have a foul odor?

If you answered "yes" to three or more of these questions, then you are experiencing the effects of an *ama* or toxin build up.

3-Day Simple Cleanse

A cleanse doesn't have to be extreme to be effective. Some extreme forms of cleansing such as water fasts, fruit juice or fruit fasts do more harm than good. They leave the body feeling sick, weak, fatigued, achy and imbalanced. Ayurveda discourages fruit fasts, or fruit juice fasts in particular, because excess sweet taste alone can actually produce toxins in the body. An excess of the sweet taste in fruit is known to dampen the digestive fire or metabolism, which is exactly the opposite of what we wish to accomplish. Fruit fasting is also inappropriate for persons with blood sugar issues such as diabetes or hypoglycemia. Eating fruit or fruit juice exclusively also creates excess acidity in the body. The body functions ideally in a more alkaline state. In Ayurveda, health is the result of balance. An Ayurvedic cleanse seeks to rebalance the body as it cleanses. Dietary extremes are unnecessary and these only create further imbalance. The following 3-day cleanse is a balancing and detoxifying cleanse. For the next 3 days we will be eliminating foods and eating habits which contain or produce *ama* or toxins.

It is important to be aware that as you begin to cleanse the body, since the brain is part of the physical body, you will notice the mind cleansing too. Thoughts, emotions, and memories may rise to the surface. If this happens, simply observe them as they arise and allow them to release. This is our first opportunity to notice the connection of body and mind. Chances are if there are toxins stored in the body, there are some mental toxins as well. There is no better time than now to release those too. When they surface, simply let them go. If tears arise, know that crying itself is a *krya* or cleansing process. Allow the cleanse to work at all levels without judgment. During and after the cleanse, you will begin to feel lighter in body, mind and spirit, as toxins are released physically and mentally. It is important to know that at any time during the next 40 days, if you feel you have come off track, simply repeat the *3-day cleanse*. I repeat the cleanse after vacation, holidays or anytime my eating habits have become derailed. For me it is like pressing a "reset button"!

Things to Avoid:

1. Junk food
2. Fast food
3. Meat/eggs
4. Desserts
5. Processed food
6. Canned food-(nutrients, quality and life-force of the food are affected)

7. Frozen dinners
8. Leftovers (no more than 24 hours) (Food begins to deteriorate and form toxins after 24 hours.)
9. Soft drinks
10. Alcohol
11. Fried food
12. White sugar
13. Artificial sweeteners
14. White flour
15. Non-organic dairy
16. Candy
17. Chewing gum (contains sugar or artificial sweeteners, also stimulates appetite)
18. Margarine and other hydrogenated fats
19. High fructose corn syrup
20. Preservatives
21. Artificial flavors and colors
22. Excessive or strenuous physical activity such as running, spinning, weight lifting, hot Yoga, power Yoga and "boot camp" classes should be avoided during the 3-day cleanse. This creates *ama* or toxins in the body. Any moderate physical activity such as Tai Chi, qigong, walking, gentle or moderate Yoga is encouraged. Taking a rest from strenuous activity allows your body to focus on detoxification.

Things to Embrace:

1. The Ayurvedic practice of beginning each morning with an 8 oz. cup of hot lemon water. Make sure the water is filtered or bottled to ensure purity. Make sure the lemon is organic. Squeeze and then drop a wedge of lemon into a mug of hot water. Include the rind since it contains many beneficial cleansing properties. Drink this before brushing teeth or ingesting any food. It is not necessary to wait longer than 10-20 minutes to eat afterwards. Since the stomach and small intestine are emptied overnight, the lemon juice is being absorbed right away. (Read below to discover the *Amazing* properties of hot lemon water.)

2. Any fresh, preferably organic, fruits, berries and vegetables, some cooked and some raw. Ex. Soups, salads, and stir-fries.

3. Nuts of all kinds—preferably organic. Peanuts, cashews and pistachio nuts should be organic due to the use of chemical pesticides on these plants.

4. Feel free to sweeten with agave nectar, molasses (highest in anti-oxidants), honey, maple syrup, raw sugar or stevia. (Maple syrup has been shown to contain 54 different beneficial mineral compounds!)

5. If you drink tea or coffee, opt for organic. Coffee and tea are often grown in countries with less strenuous regulations on harmful pesticides. I suggest you try a detoxifying tea. (See recipe at end of chapter.)

6. Feel free to use oils, such as olive, sesame, flaxseed, coconut, pumpkin, walnut, sunflower, grape seed or hempseed . . . Organic is best.

7. Enjoy cooking with Ayurvedic spices such as fresh ginger, cinnamon, cardamom, turmeric, cayenne, or black pepper. These spices help the body detoxify.

8. Enjoy any whole grains, such as whole wheat, quinoa, brown rice, black rice (highest in antioxidants), faro, barley, whole grain oats, oatmeal, or millet. (Preferably organic when available.) Season these with oils, spices, sea salt, etc. Get creative and add vegetables, nuts and berries!

9. Before eating again after a meal, allow the meal to fully digest for 3 to 4 hours. According to Ayurveda, eating again before the previous meal has been digested creates *ama* or toxins, and taxes the digestive system. It is also said to cool the digestive fire or *agni*, thus slowing the metabolism. Eating again before the meal is fully digested, places undigested food on top of partially digested food, called *chyme* in the Ayurvedic system, slowing digestion and metabolism. Personally, this principal alone made an enormous difference. It helped me to realize how much I was eating between meals when I wasn't even hungry! This principle helped me to realize what a "grazer" I was, and it helped stop me in my tracks when I found myself searching the pantry or refrigerator an hour after finishing my last meal!

10. Organic 70% cacao dark chocolate. Organic because chocolate is an imported food and is often brought from countries with less stringent pesticide regulations. Dark because milk chocolate contains high amounts of white sugar. Having chocolate on hand during the cleanse can help you make it through times of temptation. During winter I recommend hot chocolate using organic low-fat milk and organic dark drinking chocolate. Dark chocolate has positive effects: increased metabolism, reduced appetite and is a powerful anti-oxidant.

11. Enjoy another cup, 8 oz., of hot lemon water during the day, between meals, and before bed. To make this concoction more palatable and to increase the detoxifying properties of lemon water, feel free to add ginger, honey, and cinnamon, all of which have detoxifying properties!

12. Do not eat right before bed or during the night. The digestive fire *agni* slows down while the body is sleeping. Food then sits longer in the gut and begins to putrefy in the intestines, forming toxins. At least 2-3 hours is recommended between eating a snack or meal and bedtime.

13. Avoid hard core or strenuous activity for the next 3 days. You body will be using extra energy to purge toxins from cells. It is important to note that excessive exercise actually produces toxins in the system! We do not want to undo the detoxifying effects of the cleanse. A gentle or restorative Yoga practice is recommended during this time!

14. Raw fruits and vegetables, fresh bitter greens such as spinach, arugula, kale, Swiss chard, dandelion greens, basil and beet greens, and heating spices such as ginger, black pepper, and cayenne, help activate and boost the detoxification process.

15. Kitchari is a simple Ayurvedic dish often used during an Ayurvedic cleanse. I have included my own Kitchari recipe variation below. Feel free to eat this dish for breakfast, lunch or dinner, or all three! Although it is not mandatory, I highly suggest that you try this dish at least once during the cleanse. A traditional Ayurvedic cleanse will actually include kitchari 3-7 days for all 3 meals. Kitchari helps cleanse and detoxify the body and at the same time keeps it in balance.

*For a quick guide to the cleanse refer to the Appendix. Feel free to tear this page out and keep it handy!

Benefits associated with the Ayurvedic practice of consumption of hot lemon water:

Daily consumption of lemon water, particularly first thing in the morning, provides enormous health benefits. Lemon is a great source of vitamin C, vitamin B, riboflavin, potassium, magnesium, calcium, and phosphorus. Beginning the day with lemon water restores pH balance in the body, rehydrates the tissues, and stimulates peristalsis. Lemon water is said to rejuvenate the skin from the inside out, act as a blood purifier and a liver tonic. Hot lemon water stimulates the body's ability to flush out toxins, and is said to be effective in reducing body weight more quickly. It lowers blood pressure, relieves asthma, and promotes a sense of relaxation, and reduces anxiety and depression. There are current studies showing evidence that lemon may have powerful anti-cancer properties, possibly more powerful than chemotherapy itself, yet lemon does not adversely affect healthy cells. In Ayurveda, hot water is said to "melt" the sludge of toxins or *ama* off the intestinal walls when taken first thing in the morning on an empty stomach. Since it also stimulates the elimination process, the toxins are then removed from the body as waste.

It is important to use only organic lemons since we are working towards detoxification. Conventionally grown citrus fruits are highly sprayed. The lemon should be squeezed into the hot water then dropped into the cup, peel and all. Many of the beneficial properties of the lemon are found in the peel!

Focus for Today: Really tune in to how you feel during "the cleanse". As your body begins to clean out toxins, the mind will begin to cleanse too. Notice if any thoughts, impressions or memories come to the surface and release. Notice if you begin to feel lighter in mind, body and spirit, as mental and physical toxins release.

Journal: Feel free to journal about the release of mental "toxins" as well as physical ones here in this space!

We will begin a Daily Food Journal today as well. You will find it on the next page. This food journal will help keep you honest with yourself, and through it you will begin to identify eating patterns which are standing in your way of optimal health, energy and vitality. (The Daily Food Journal was inspired by dear friend Becky DeAmaco and developed and designed by dear friend and Enlightened Eating student Shannon Schomberg.)

Recipes of the Day:

Elise's Simple Kitchari Recipe

This is a traditional Ayurvedic cleansing dish. (Use organic ingredients as much as possible. Most of the ingredients have cleansing properties. It is traditionally served over Basmati rice. I also sometimes enjoy it with quinoa. It can be made in the Crockpot on low.

1 cup split mung beans (red lentils can be substituted, however mung beans have powerful detoxifying properties, and are balancing for all constitutions, lentils are not.
1 carrot, finely chopped
3 ½ to 4 cups water (I use filtered water)
2 tbsp extra virgin olive oil
1 tsp turmeric
½ tsp cardamom
½ tsp coriander
1 piece of ginger, finely chopped,
about the size of the top of the thumb
Large handful of fresh cilantro, chopped
¼ tsp cumin
1 small bay leaf
3 cloves garlic minced
2 cups fresh organic spinach, chard or kale (bitter greens)
Juice of ½ lemon
Sea salt and pepper to taste

Although it is not necessary, I soak the beans for at least 3 hours prior to cooking them. First, heat the dry spices in the olive oil until fragrant. Stir in the carrots, garlic, ginger and allow to soften. Add mung beans and water to mixture. Reduce heat and allow to thicken so that it is no longer watery, which is about 45 minutes. Add the cilantro, spinach and lemon juice, at the end and cook until spinach and cilantro are wilted. Salt and pepper to taste. Serve over organic brown basmati rice or organic quinoa.

Detoxifying Tea

Here is a recipe for "Detoxifying Tea" from The Council of Maharishi Ayurveda Physicians:

Boil two quarts of water in the morning.
Add ¼ tsp. cumin
½ tsp. coriander
½ tsp. fennel seed

Add the spices to the water and let steep for ten minutes with the lid on.
Strain out the spices and pour the water into a thermos.
Sip throughout the day.
Make a new batch of tea every morning.

Daily Food Journal

Date:_____   Intention for the day:_____   Weight:_____

Water: *X off one water for every 8 oz. of water that you drink. This includes lemon waters. During a cleanse you should have at least 3 lemon waters daily.*

YOGI PLATE ➡   ¼ Protein ➡   ½ Veggies
                 ¼ Whole Grains ➡

Rate your hunger, mood, energy

and after meal satisfaction

| 1=Low | 2=Average | 3=High |

Time	Meal/ Snack	Food/ Beverage	Hungry?	Mood?	Energy?	Satisfied?
	Breakfast					
	Snack					
	Lunch					
	Snack					
	Dinner					
	Snack					

At the end of the day, reflect on how many servings you had of the following foods/beverages:

Food	Servings
Vegetables (Unlimited)	
Whole Grains (Women 1 -3)	
Fruit (Aim for 2)	
Protein (Aim for 3 or more)	

Did I Avoid?	Yes	No	How Much?
Alcohol			
Soft Drinks			
White Sugar			
Artificial Sweeteners			
Processed Food			
Fast Food			

Alert! Use Meat Sparingly

Consume meat no more than 3 times a week!

List your observations and insights for the day. These include successes and behaviors that need attention:

_____
_____
_____
_____
_____

Day 3: Setting Intentions

"Intentions compressed into words enfold magical power." ~Deepak Chopra

Sankalpa is the Sanskrit word for intention. Intention is defined as a sustained or unbroken commitment or purpose. The practice of setting intentions is potent, even magical. We unconsciously set intentions all the time. "This organic cookie isn't going to taste good." "I must have dessert every night." A few weeks ago I was meeting a friend for lunch after a meditation class. That morning she said, "I bet your stomach will growl when you're trying to meditate, anticipating our lunch." Guess what happened . . . I think the whole room could hear my stomach growling.

Other people can set intentions for you, if you let them! During the Enlightened Eating classes I conduct, almost every student shares how friends and family members try to derail their new way of eating. Other people may try to override your intentions with their own intentions, and they will if you allow it. My students have received intention setting comments from family, friends and co-workers like "You're never going to be able to go through with this." or "You have no will-power." Others may try to set their intentions for you in the form of tempting. One group member had a neighbor bring over an ice cream pie during the 3-day cleanse. She sat and watched as her family ate the pie, but noted later that she actually felt empowered by keeping her own intentions. Another group member had friends wave tempting foods under her nose at a party in an effort to foil her resolve. She too was able to allow the power of her own intentions to prevail over her friends' less than noble temptations. Group members have also taken flack from co-workers for their new way of eating. Co-workers have brought baked goods into the office in order to entice enlightened eaters away from their new found path. At home, it is not uncommon for children to snub new foods, and complain at meals that there is nothing they like. Spouses seem to attempt to challenge intentions the most. One group member's husband took up baking enticing breads just as she had resolved to change her eating in order to improve her health. Other spouses complained that their partner wasn't as fun as before they changed their eating, or called them "high maintenance."

Be aware that others will try and thwart your intentions over the next 40 days. Other people may try to overpower your intentions with their own. Often these intentions are not righteous in nature. It is said that misery loves company. Seeing someone else improve their weight and health shines an uncomfortable light on their own weight and health. With friends, coworkers and spouses, sometimes the green eyed monster comes out to play. Perhaps they are worried that you will look better than they do, or be more attractive to the opposite sex. Frequently, friends and spouses are afraid that if you look better and feel better, you may no longer be the same person that they know and love. Of course what happens in reality is that you are the same person, only better!

It is important to let those around you know of your intentions. Ask them to support you during the 40 days. Challenge them to join you on the 40 day journey or just enlist them to help you stay on track, and tell them you truly need their help. Do not let anyone else set intentions for you but you. You alone know what you need, and you alone know what is best for you. You have a right to look, feel and think your best.

Whether we're aware of it or not, the choices we make regarding the foods we eat are setting intentions for our health, our weight, our energy, vitality and youthfulness. I have a relative who drinks six to twelve diet Mountain Dews a day. This is certainly setting intentions for her health. Her *body* knows she is not drinking "dew" from a mountain!

The compelling thing is we have the power consciously to determine our own intentions. We can use intention "intentionally" to reinforce and strengthen our goals. When intentions are set, the mind becomes focused on them. Where the mind focuses, energy follows. Where energy flows, action results. Now we are going to set our own intentions from the start. We will harness the power of intention to create new healthier patterns of eating and living. Setting intentions is often compared to planting seeds. When these seeds are placed in fertile soil they sprout and grow, blossoming forth into what they are destined to become.

Breakfast is the meal that sets our eating intentions for the day. Skipping breakfast sets the intent of starving the body and the brain. The body will quickly rebel, and kick out hormones that will induce a ravenous appetite impossible to resist as the day wears on. Eating an unhealthy breakfast, such as drinking a diet soda, eating a pastry or slice of cake, also sets the tone for the day. It says, "I've already blown it! What is the point of trying to eat right the rest of the day?"

By making healthful breakfast choices, you are setting the intention of feeling energized, balanced, and nourished for the rest of the day. Making a yummy, yet nutritious choice for breakfast means that you are setting the intention for how you are going to eat that day. Setting your intentions for the 40 day journey sets into motion a new way of feeling, living and being.

A Chinese saying:

From intention springs the deed,
From the deed springs the habits,
From the habits grows the character,
From the character develops the destiny.

Focus for Today:

1. By selecting a tasty yet nutritious breakfast, you are setting your intentions today. Try one of the breakfast suggestions listed under Recipes of the Day! Let your lemon water and breakfast choices set your intentions each day for the 40 days and beyond!

2. Set your intentions to be successful over the next 40 days by cleaning out your cupboards, pantry, refrigerator, and freezer of all processed foods, junk foods and foods containing artificial chemicals, preservatives, additives, colors, and flavors. Rid your home of sodas, hydrogenated oils and artificial sweeteners. Set your intentions to eat real foods divinely created (not man-made) to optimally nourish and strengthen the mind-body system. Fresh, whole foods do not create toxins in the system which slow down digestion, metabolism, and promote premature aging. Set your intentions to toss out things that haven't been working in your favor to bring forth health, youthfulness and vitality.

3. Appendix 1 contains a grocery list of suggested healthy foods. This will help you replace all the foods which have been discarded. Keeping foods which don't honor your body or your health also sets intentions. It sets the intention that you are not making a true and permanent change. It sets the intention that you will go back to this way of eating in time. It sets the intention that you will not follow through with the 40 days! Be aware of this intention too, and be aware that intentions are extremely powerful.

4. Clear your closet of your "fat clothes", clothes which no longer fit, but which you are keeping just in case you gain weight. Keeping these items sets an intention that you will wear them again. Set the intention that they will never fit again and donate them or give them away!

Journal: What are the reasons you began this 40 day journey? What is it you would like to result from the next 40 days? Consider what intentions you have been unconsciously setting (positive or negative). For example, smoking a pack a day sets an intention about your health, as does drinking six Diet Mountain Dews a day.

Write down your intentions for the next 40 days. Make sure you word your intentions in a positive way. Write them again in the present tense, as if you've already succeeded. For example," I have successfully dropped four dress sizes, my energy is through the roof, and I look and feel the best I ever have!" Sitting in a quiet state of awareness, visualize yourself having already succeeded in accomplishing these intentions. Post your written intentions in a place where you will see it often, and read it to yourself every day.

Recipes of the Day:

Let these healthy suggestions inspire you to create breakfasts which set the intention of how you plan to eat for the whole day!

Breakfast Berry Smoothie

(Serves 1)
1 cup organic Greek yogurt (low-fat)
1 cup frozen mixed berries, blueberries, strawberries or raspberries (organic if possible)
½ cup filtered water
1-2 Tbsp organic agave nectar (to taste, depending on the sweetness of the berries)

Blend thoroughly in blender.

Quick and Easy Cashew-Cinnamon Smoothie

(Serves 1)
2 Tbsp cashew butter or ½ cup cashews
¼ tsp cinnamon
6 oz water
¼ to ½ tsp agave nectar (to desired sweetness)

Blend together until smooth. Heat and enjoy as a warm drink if desired.

Mango-Cinnamon Smoothie

(Serves 1)

½ mango, chopped into large cubes
¾ cup low-fat organic Greek yogurt
4 oz water
1-2 tsp agave nectar
¼ tsp cinnamon

Blend together thoroughly in blender.

Enlightened Chocolate Peanut Butter Smoothie

(Serves 1)

1 heaping Tbsp organic peanut butter
3 heaping Tbsp cocoa powder
1-2 tsp organic agave nectar
8oz purified water

Blend the above ingredients in blender. Use hot water during fall or winter if you prefer a warm smoothie!

Enlightened Pina Colada Smoothie

(Serves 1)

½ cup fresh pineapple pieces
4 oz light coconut milk
½ cup low fat organic Greek yogurt
¼ cup unsweetened shredded coconut

Blend together in blender . . . Enjoy!

Oatmeal Recipe 1: Organic oatmeal sweetened with maple syrup, walnuts, and apple slices, and or white raisins.

Oatmeal Recipe 2: Oatmeal with pumpkin seeds, cinnamon and dried figs, sweetened with agave nectar.

Oatmeal Recipe 3: Oatmeal with dried cranberries, peanuts, or any other nut, and cinnamon.

Oatmeal Tip:

Put steel cut oats in your Crockpot before you go to bed and wake up to a good intention! Try adding dried cherries, fresh apple pieces, white raisins, walnuts, pecans, almonds, pumpkin seeds, coconut, cinnamon, or nutmeg. Top with a splash of almond, coconut or soy milk, and drizzle with maple syrup. Use 1 cup steel cut oats to 3 cups of water . . . place Crockpot on lowest setting.

Other Breakfast Ideas:

Fruit and whole grain toast.

Nut butters on whole grain or sprouted toast drizzled with honey and sprinkled with cinnamon

Greek yogurt topped with organic granola

Other whole grain cereal such as quinoa, with added fruit or nuts

Natural fruit and nut bars such as Kind bars, Lara bars, Pro-bars, or Bora Bora bars

Toast sprouted cinnamon raisin bread, top with butter or ghee, serve with a glass of fresh squeezed grapefruit juice.

Daily Food Journal

Date:_____   Intention for the day:_____   Weight:_____

Water: 🔲🔲🔲🔳🔳🔳🔳   *X off one water for every 8 oz. of water that you drink. This includes lemon waters. During a cleanse you should have at least 3 lemon waters daily.*

YOGI PLATE →	¼ Protein ¼ Whole Grains →	→ ½ Veggies

Rate your hunger, mood, energy
and after meal satisfaction

1=Low	2=Average	3=High

Time	Meal/ Snack	Food/ Beverage	Hungry?	Mood?	Energy?	Satisfied?
	Breakfast					
	Snack					
	Lunch					
	Snack					
	Dinner					
	Snack					

At the end of the day, reflect on how many servings you had of the following foods/beverages:

Vegetables (Unlimited)	
Whole Grains (Women 1 -3)	
Fruit (Aim for 2)	
Protein (Aim for 3 or more)	

Did I Avoid?	Yes	No	How Much?
Alcohol			
Soft Drinks			
White Sugar			
Artificial Sweeteners			
Processed Food			
Fast Food			

Alert! Use Meat Sparingly
Consume meat no more than 3 times a week!

List your observations and insights for the day. These include successes and behaviors that need attention:
_____
_____
_____
_____
_____

Day 4: *Tapas*—The Fire of Transformation

"Opportunities to find deeper powers within ourselves come when life seems most challenging." ~Joseph Campbell

Tapas is a Sanskrit word, literally meaning "heat" or "to burn". It loosely translates as self-discipline, enthusiasm, and excitement. *Tapas* is about tapping into your "inner fire", your innermost drive, and your "burning desire" to become the ideal you. *Tapas* is "focused effort", self-discipline and restraint, in order to achieve a higher purpose. *Tapas* is a Yoga concept that can be applied to any aspect of your life. For example, it takes *tapas* to dedicate yourself to practice the piano until one day you are able to play the most complex concertos. The same can be said when it comes to eating and food. Without the inner drive and "burning desire" to live a life thriving with health, energy and longevity, right eating will not happen. It takes *tapas*, an "inner burning" for achieving your best self, to make intention a reality. It takes *tapas* at each meal and each snack to eat in a disciplined way, a way that is in alignment with your intention for the 40 days. *Tapas* is a concept in which the "fire of discipline" out-burns the craving for wrong foods. It is a discipline that must be practiced with constant attention and awareness. It is making the commitment to taking each step necessary on an ongoing basis to achieve that which you desire. *Tapas* is the discipline it takes for each eating choice you make to lead you one step closer to optimal weight, energy, health and vitality.

Tapas is the fire of transformation. It gives us the intensity to burn away that which no longer serves us and that which overshadows our true brilliance. When gold is placed in the fire, the impurities are burned away, and its beauty and radiance are revealed. When we let our burning desire for change power us through the "impurities" of eating temptations, we come away more pure in mind, body and spirit. When we allow the fire of discipline that is *tapas* help us transform our old ways of eating into something new and healthier, like the gold, we too will emerge from the fire radiating with beauty, and luminous with health.

Tapas is not forced, but it is self-imposed discipline. It is voluntarily engaging in a practice which will precipitate self-change. As we practice the steady and focused discipline it takes to eat whole natural foods consistently, in place of foods which do not serve us, we do so knowing that a better self will emerge. *Tapas* is a self-discipline that retrains the mind. The word *tapas* actually comes from the ancient word *tapasvin*, an original name given to someone who practiced Yoga. *Tapasvin* refers to someone who practices voluntary self-control and willing restraint in order to "burn away" undesired qualities which stand in the way of achieving a higher intention. (A Yoga mat was originally called a *tapas* mat.) *Tapas* in eating is voluntary self-restraint, knowing the results of this practice will be the fulfillment of the intentions you have set for this 40 days. Know that this voluntary restraint will re-train the mind to make better eating choices on an ongoing basis.

In Yogic texts, the mind-body system is likened to wild horses pulling a chariot. The mind is the wild horses. The body is the chariot. The chariot driver holding the reins is the will or intellect. If the wild horses are left to control the chariot without being reined in by the driver, the result is chaos and disharmony along the journey, with the horses confused and running in all different directions. This would make it impossible to reach the destination. It is necessary for the driver to firmly control the reins and discipline the horses in order for him to reach his destination. We must rely then on the intellect to "rein-in" and discipline our chaotic minds. Our minds are often off and running in various directions controlled by impulsive reactions to our senses when it comes to eating and food. We often lack control. It is *tapas* which gives us the "fire" to keep the mind in check, when it comes to how and what we eat.

Along our 40 day journey to Enlightened Eating, it is important for us to tap into that inner burning to become our best self. We can "harness" that inner desire to help us rein in old, unproductive eating tendencies and habits, so that we can transform along the journey, and arrive at our desired destination. It is in the moments when temptation presents itself, and your will is able to prevail, when transformation happens and old patterns and habits are burned away. *Tapas* is the fire of determination which ultimately results in transformation.

"Perseverance is the path to transformation." ~Elise Cantrell

Focus for Today: Find a burning desire to see these 40 days through. Delve into your own inner fire to burn away doubts and fear of change. Let the fire of *tapas* drive you to stay committed to this 40-day process. Let your focused effort lead you to meet your best-self at the end of this journey. Let your inner fire "burn away" that which doesn't serve you.

Journal: List eating habits that you've had in the past that do not serve you. List concrete behaviors you plan to enact in order to "rein in" these unproductive patterns now and after the 40 days. Practice these new behaviors. This is your *tapas,* your own individualized practice or self-imposed discipline. This practice is intended to result in positive change, in this case, the best you.

Recipe of the Day:

Bananas Foster with Vanilla Crème

(Serves 4)

4 ripe bananas
3 Tbsp butter
½ tsp cinnamon
1 Tbsp brown sugar
1 container vanilla Greek yogurt

Slice bananas in half. Melt butter in skillet. Add bananas, sugar and cinnamon. Cook until caramelized. Blend vanilla yogurt until liquefied. Place caramelized bananas on dessert plate and drizzle with liquefied yogurt.

Daily Food Journal

Date:_____ Intention for the day:_____ Weight:_____

Water: ⬜⬜⬜⬛⬛⬛⬛⬛ *X off one water for every 8 oz. of water that you drink. This includes lemon waters. During a cleanse you should have at least 3 lemon waters daily.*

YOGI PLATE ➡

¼ Protein
½ Veggies
¼ Whole Grains

Rate your hunger, mood, energy and after meal satisfaction

| 1=Low | 2=Average | 3=High |

Time	Meal/Snack	Food/Beverage	Hungry?	Mood?	Energy?	Satisfied?
	Breakfast					
	Snack					
	Lunch					
	Snack					
	Dinner					
	Snack					

At the end of the day, reflect on how many servings you had of the following foods/beverages:

Vegetables (Unlimited)	
Whole Grains (Women 1 -3)	
Fruit (Aim for 2)	
Protein (Aim for 3 or more)	

Did I Avoid?	Yes	No	How Much?
Alcohol			
Soft Drinks			
White Sugar			
Artificial Sweeteners			
Processed Food			
Fast Food			

Alert! Use Meat Sparingly

Consume meat no more than 3 times a week!

List your observations and insights for the day. These include successes and behaviors that need attention:

_____
_____
_____
_____
_____

Phase 1: Food and the Body

Now that we have opened our minds, cleansed our systems, set our intentions, and stoked the flames of *tapas*, the first phase of "Enlightened Eating" begins with food and the body. We will gain new insights when it comes to our physical body and the way we eat. We will learn new ways of eating and gain new perspectives about food in order to optimize how we look and feel in our physical body!

"Even in favorable conditions, a person encounters struggle."
~Swami Kripalu

You may have begun to notice resistance. Struggle and frustration may begin to arise as you are sticking with the plan. You may have noticed drops in mood and energy at this point. This is because our bodies have become conditioned (sometimes for decades) to having simple carbs and processed foods for quick energy and mood pick-me-ups, and now your body is no longer getting them. The "withdrawal" is beginning. The key is to be aware that this is what is happening! The BIG key is to be bigger than the cravings that you are experiencing! This is when it gets tougher, but transformation is beginning! Once you break through the barrier of using the wrong foods to solve sluggish energy and low moods, your mood and energy will begin to stabilize simply by eating the right foods consistently. Cravings will diminish. However, you have to get through this trying stage to move beyond the strong desire for the wrong foods. Enlightened Eating is about resetting the cravings and the appetite for nourishing foods rather than using food as a "drug" for quick energy and mood enhancement. In emergencies, remember organic dark chocolate is in the plan, and eating just a few squares can be helpful in a pinch. Dark chocolate is reputed to have some metabolic boosting benefits. I also recommend calming teas. Kava tea is my favorite! I suggest finding strategies other than food to perk up energy. There is nothing like fresh air and sunshine! Do something to distract yourself when cravings hit . . . and the cravings will pass! Practice just observing moments of weakness and cravings as they arise, and allow them to go by without reacting to them. Those cravings are the "wild horses" you read about yesterday. It is time for your will or intellect to take the reins, and guide the wild horses that are the food cravings in the right direction . . . to optimal health, weight, mood and energy!

Now that we have completed the cleanse, we are able to begin adding foods back into our diet carefully, and with awareness. Take notice of how you feel during and after eating certain foods. Restock your home with fresh, whole foods, whole grains, fruits and vegetables. Purchase flavorful teas, natural sweeteners, and lots of organic lemons! Each day, set your intentions for the day with the breakfast you choose. By making a healthy nutritious choice for breakfast, you will be amazed at how the rest of the day falls into place. By making a disastrous choice for breakfast, you will be shocked at how the rest of the day falls apart! We will be continuing to document our eating in the Enlightened Eating "Daily Food Journal".

Food Do's Phase 1:

1. Drink 8 oz. warm lemon water each morning before anything else is ingested. It is no longer necessary to drink it throughout the day. Make sure you are using fresh organic lemons, not bottled lemon juice. Put the slices into the water, because some of the active enzymes and essential oils are in the peel. The heat releases these into the water. Also, because the lemon is fresh, there are more active properties in the lemon slices. This is an Ayurvedic daily practice or *dynacharya* for optimal health. It is highly recommended that you continue this practice well beyond the 40 Days. Make this a practice for life! Surprisingly, lemon water is alkalinizing to the body making it less hospitable to disease.

2. Coffee should be organic. Teas should be organic when possible.

3. Let your breakfast set the intentions for your eating each day by choosing a delicious, nourishing and healthful breakfast.

4. Continue eating a mix of raw and cooked organic fruits and vegetables. Soups, salads, stir-fries are all great options.

5. All breads should be 100% whole grain. Organic sprouted breads are ideal.

6. Chocolate should be organic 70% cocoa.

7. Enjoy nuts and nut butters. Peanut butter should be organic.

8. Use oils such as sesame, olive, coconut, flaxseed, pumpkin, walnut, sunflower, grape seed, hempseed, organic butter, or "*ghee*", which is clarified butter. The recipe for *ghee* is included in this chapter. *Ghee* is said to be an ideal food and have powerful Ayurvedic healing properties. In Ayurveda, *ghee* is used as a medicine and it is also mixed with herbs, used as a vehicle to transport the herbs to the bodily tissues.

9. Continue to use whole grains and nutrient-dense brown rice and whole grain pastas.

10. Continue to wait until a meal is fully digested before eating again or snacking. Wait 3-4 hours, and continue to avoid eating right before bed. When we add un-digested food to partially digested food, we diminish the digestive fire. This slows the digestive process and creates *ama*. This slows the metabolism.

11. Portion your plate as follows. A Yogi's plate consists of:

    ¼ protein
    ¼ grains
    ½ fresh vegetables and fruits, cooked or raw.
    Your entire meal should be able to fit in the palms of both hands cupped together. A quantity of food greater than this will weaken the digestive fire, creating toxins.

12. Meats should be free-range, grass-fed if they are your protein. Eggs should be cage-free/organic. If you notice that you are not craving meats, do not be in a hurry to add them back. Wait until you really want them. Limit meat to three times a week. Keep in that mind nuts, dairy, soy, whole grains and legumes are healthier sources of protein.

13. Dairy is preferably organic if it is in your budget. Especially high fat dairy such as butter, cream and cheese. Hormone and antibiotic-free, grass-fed dairy is in keeping with a healthy Ayurvedic diet. Dairy products coming from farms using these practices are also acceptable. Amish farmers pride themselves in their traditional farming practices. French cheeses and butters for the most part also employ safe traditional dairy farming methods as well. Amish and French cheeses and butters are also good options. My enlightened eating students have been astonished by how quickly skin blemishes and acne disappear simply by switching to organic dairy.

14. Some suggested non-meat proteins include nuts and beans. I put both on a salad, which is delicious! I recommend sprinkling black beans, black eye peas, cashews, chickpeas, walnuts and sunflower seeds on salads. I use Greek yogurt for protein too. It is very high in protein! I make salad dressings with it, smoothies, and eat it as a snack! Tofu is high in soy protein. You can make salad dressing with tofu, or I will sometimes chop it up and put it on a salad too. Some people marinate and grill it! Nut butters on toast are great. Try cashew butter or almond butter on toast, drizzle it with raw honey and sprinkle a little cinnamon on top! It is yummy! I make smoothies with nut butters too, and some of those recipes are included in Chapter 3. Hummus with baked, whole grain pita chips is a protein-filled treat! Whole grains have a lot of protein too, such as oatmeal and brown rice. Quinoa has the highest protein levels of all grains, so you can get plenty of protein without ever eating meat!

15. Desserts, if any, should be mostly fruit-based (fresh, cooked or raw), and should not be sweetened with white sugar or artificial sweeteners. Natural sweeteners and spices are fine.

16. Give yourself at least 2-3 hours for your food to digest before you go to sleep.

17. Drink plenty of fresh pure water. This helps your body continue to flush out toxins. Feel free to flavor your water with natural juices, herbs, etc. to make it more enjoyable. You will notice the Daily Food Journal has a section in which each 8oz. of water you drink is X-ed out. Try to X out all of the water glasses each day!

Food Don'ts Phase 1:

1. Do not drink iced beverages. Ice cold drinks cool the digestive fire. Slowing the digestive fire slows the metabolism. Beverages can be warm, cool or room temperature.

2. Do not eat meat more than three times this week. Meat is difficult to digest and creates *ama* in the body as it putrefies during the digestive process. Meat is also higher on the food chain and contains more toxins, especially factory farmed meat. If you are not craving meat, then wait to add it back into your diet until you are actually "craving" it. I encourage you to use grass-fed, free-range meat because it contains fewer toxins and more nutrients. Since you are eating less meat, this should not affect your budget. (See appendix "10 Ways to Save Money by Eating Healthy.") Eat fish and seafood no more than twice weekly, due to toxic contaminants found in fish.

3. Avoid microwaving foods whenever possible. According to Ayurveda, microwaves damage foods' life-force. In studies more nutrients are destroyed through microwave heating than through other forms of heating. Avoid aluminum cookware which is said to impart toxic properties into the food according to Ayurvedic texts. It is preferable to cook with copper or clay based cookware. Avoid cookware with non-stick coatings which have been shown to release toxins into the food.

4. No processed food, junk food, fast food, or deep-fried food. These contain *ama*. The 3-day cleanse has begun to rid the system of toxins. In order to optimize the metabolism, it is important to limit toxins entering the system. It is important to understand that when we introduce toxins into the system, the metabolism becomes sluggish as it attempts to process aberrant foods.

5. No artificial sweeteners or white sugar. According to Ayurveda, white sugar increases *ama* in the body. White sugar is said to weaken the immune system and feed infections. Sweetness itself is not something to avoid and is not forbidden in the Enlightened Eating plan. Opt for natural sweeteners such as raw honey, stevia, agave,

molasses, maple syrup, or raw sugar. If you find that you regularly have strong cravings for sweets, it may be a sign that you are actually craving for more "sweetness" in your life. To reduce these cravings, add more "sweetness" into your living rather than into your eating.

6. No artificial ingredients. Rule of thumb: if it sounds like a chemical or you can't pronounce it, don't eat it. It's not "really" food.

7. Limit alcoholic beverages to red wine which actually has beneficial anti-inflammatory and anti-oxidant properties. Women, no more than 1 glass/day; men no more than 2 glasses/day. Overconsumption of alcohol creates *ama*. If you notice that wine creates a toxic effect for you, then it should be eliminated entirely. I have found organic and sulfite-free wines have the fewest toxic effects (joint discomfort, puffiness, water-retention, inflammation, fatigue) on my own body. Therefore, I recommend drinking organic wine if alcohol is a must.

8. Avoid left-overs older than 24 hours, or re-heated foods when possible. These foods have begun to loose *prana* or life-force, and accumulate bacteria and toxins. I recommend freezing left-overs which you do not plan to eat within 24 hours. It then becomes a convenient meal on a busy day.

9. No soft drinks, candy or gum.

10. No margarine, only real butter, *ghee* or natural oils (nothing hydrogenated).

11. I have provided a "suggested" grocery list in the Appendix to help you with ideas to navigate the 40 Days. In no way is this list a must by any means, but is meant to be a resource to help you as you shop. I suggest going to the store when you can really take time to read ingredients and discover new products which will truly serve you along the 40 day journey.

12. There is no "blowing it," there is no "giving up". At anytime during the 40 day journey when you find you have strayed from the path to enlighten eating, simply repeat the 3-Day Cleanse. I find with my students that just about everyone has a point in which they have become derailed from eating the right foods. With Enlightened Eating if we discover

this has happened, we simply repeat the cleanse and keep moving ahead! We never get lost or left behind. Giving up simply isn't an option.

Focus for Phase 1: For the first segment of the plan, we will primarily focus on food and eating as it affects the body. From now through Day 21 we will be gaining new insights from Yoga and Ayurveda and my own life experience and research on how what we eat impacts the body. Each day is a step towards transformation and a step closer to your ideal self.

Journal: Note any interesting insights in your journal throughout the week. What are you craving? Why? Be sure to document what you are eating in your daily food journal, and note how it makes you feel!

Recipe for Phase 1:

How to Make Ghee

1 lb. unsalted organic butter

Melt the butter in a saucepan over medium heat and bring to boil, stirring.
Let the butter simmer gently for 15 minutes.

Remove the pan from the heat. Do not remove the foam at the top due to its medicinal properties.
Allow the *ghee* to cool for about 2 hours.

Strain the *ghee* into a glass jar. I prefer a fine wire strainer but traditionally cheese cloth is used.

The jar of *ghee* can be kept unrefrigerated in a dark cabinet for up to 6 months.

Day 5: You Really Are What You Eat!

"Tell me what you eat, and I'll tell you what you are." During the Age of Enlightenment, this declaration was made by renowned French gastronomist Jean Anthelme Brillat-Savarin. This statement marked the foundation of the science of eating and food here in the west. His book acknowledged how preparing, cooking, and eating foods affects the whole human. He asserted that it was food which was the "measure of strength and prosperity of whole empires." This philosophy was new to the west at this time, but it has actually been a part of the science of Ayurveda for 5000 years. In Ayurveda, the physical body is referred to as the *annamaya kosha*, or "food sheath". The physical body and the mind are said to be composed solely of the things we ingest. If you're ingesting fresh foods filled with nutrients, energy and vitality, then your body, skin, hair and nails will look and feel nourished and vital. Your mind will be clear and sharp.

If you are eating artificial or processed foods devoid of life and nutrients, your physical body and mental nature will reflect that energy. Simple physical tasks such as walking or climbing stairs can become a challenge. The skin, hair, and nails aren't vibrant; the immune system does not function at its optimal level. The body may appear bloated, and body fat may accumulate disproportionally in the belly, thighs, hips, back of the arms, face, chin and/or neck. Energy is low or non-existent, and the mind is sluggish. This is a portrait of someone lacking vitality. How the body feels physically directly reflects how the mind and spirit feel too. When the body is sluggish, the mind and spirit are sluggish. It is difficult to think, focus and concentrate. Energy levels and moods are low and erratic. Our spiritual connection becomes clouded, and lazy. When the body feels healthy, vital and nourished, the mind is clear and the spirit thrives. A Zen saying is: *"When the mind is clear, everything is clear; and when the mind is not clear; everything is not clear."*

With this in mind, it is important to be aware that it takes time for the body to adjust to a new way of eating. Even if the new way of eating is much healthier and cleaner, the body still must adapt to the changes because it actually becomes habituated to an imbalanced diet. Often, there can be side-effects as the body works to restore homeostasis. People who have had a previous diet containing heavy amounts of processed food, junk food, or sugary treats may even experience symptoms similar to drug withdrawal. Know that this is temporary, and as your body adjusts to new eating habits, the symptoms will subside, and better health and harmony will follow. Your system will begin to thrive in its new-normal.

Knowing that you really are what you eat can actually be empowering! It means that by changing what you eat, you can change who you are for the better and forever! The cells in the body are composed of the foods we eat. Cells are constantly being replaced at a rate of millions per second! Different cells are replaced at different speeds. For example, the lining of the stomach and the small intestine are completely replaced in less than a week. Red blood cells and the skeleton are completely replaced in 3 months. Skin cells are constantly renewing. In 1 year a large percentage of the body is completely new. In 7-10 years, 98% of the body is completely new. As we age, cells are renewed at an increasingly slower rate, but the body does continue to renew and rebuild itself every day. It is up to us to oversee how well these cells are built. You are the builder of your own body and your own health simply by the food choices that you make! Choosing the healthiest foods builds the strongest, healthiest cells.

I remember when we put an addition on our house several years ago. The builder carefully inspected each delivery of wood. Often he sent pieces of lumber back to the lumber yard because he felt the quality didn't measure up. Because of his careful attention, I feel confident our addition was well built! How much more important it is to make sure the foods we put in our body measure up so that each addition of new cells are well built too!

Focus for Today: Remember ... *"Your physical body is a representation of your past and not of your future."* ~Laura Toolin

Journal: How do you think your eating has affected your physical body? Describe what you see in the mirror. What do you think contributed to these effects? How have the things you have been eating affected your mind? What are some things you would like to see change in the mirror with a new approach to eating? What are some mental qualities you would like to see change as a result of eating?

Recipe of the Day:

Cherry Tomato / Basil Pasta

I came up with this as an answer to abundant cherry tomatoes and basil! This is quick, easy and delicious!

1 lb pasta of your choice (I use spaghetti or bow tie pasta) organic whole grain if possible
3 Tbsp olive oil
1 lb cherry tomatoes halved or quartered (depending on size)
1/2 head of garlic peeled and finely chopped
Handful of fresh basil torn into shreds
½ of 6 oz can organic tomato paste
salt
pepper

While boiling the pasta in salted water, begin to sauté the garlic, basil, and tomatoes in olive oil. When softened, add tomato paste and 3 soup ladles of salty pasta water.

The starch from the pasta will thicken the cherry tomato mixture. Just before the pasta is al-dente, remove from water and add the pasta to the tomato mixture in the sauté pan. Cook 1 more minute, it will thicken.

Serve with more torn basil and freshly grated parmesan on top!

Daily Food Journal

Date:_____   Intention for the day:_____   Weight:_____

Water: ⬜⬜⬜⬛⬛⬛⬛ X off one water for every 8 oz. of water that you drink. This includes lemon waters. During a cleanse you should have at least 3 lemon waters daily.

YOGI PLATE ➡   ¼ Protein ➡   ⬅ ½ Veggies
¼ Whole Grains ➡

| Rate your hunger, mood, energy |
| and after meal satisfaction |
| 1=Low   2=Average   3=High |

Time	Meal/ Snack	Food/ Beverage	Hungry?	Mood?	Energy?	Satisfied?
	Breakfast					
	Snack					
	Lunch					
	Snack					
	Dinner					
	Snack					

At the end of the day, reflect on how many
servings you had of the following foods/beverages:

Vegetables (Unlimited)	
Whole Grains (Women 1 -3)	
Fruit (Aim for 2)	
Protein (Aim for 3 or more)	

Did I Avoid?	Yes	No	How Much?
Alcohol			
Soft Drinks			
White Sugar			
Artificial Sweeteners			
Processed Food			
Fast Food			

| **Alert! Use Meat Sparingly** |
| Consume meat no more than 3 times a week! |

List your observations and insights for the day. These include successes and behaviors that need attention:
_____
_____
_____
_____
_____

Day 6: What is Your Eating Style?

"What you are aware of, you are in control of; what you are not aware of is in control of you." ~Anthony de Mello

Whether we are aware of it or not, we each have our own eating style. This is no different than our having our own style of dressing or decorating our home. How we eat, dress, or decorate reflects who we are. However, our habitual way of eating has a powerful influence on how we look and feel. Over our lifetime, each of us has developed our own eating style which is responsible for balance or imbalance in many other aspects of health and life. Most people never make the connection that it is their eating style which is an obstacle to looking and feeling their best. You approach to eating can have an equally significant affect as the actual food you are eating! In order to recognize whether your eating style is sabotaging your efforts to achieve optimal weight, energy, health and vitality, I have created a quiz inspired by Dr. Susan Albers' book <u>Eating Mindfully</u> and Ayurvedic eating philosophy. Awareness is the first step towards correcting an approach that is not working in your favor. Discover your eating style and how it is affecting you!

Quiz—Determine Your Eating Style:

Directions: Circle the answer to each question which best represents your way of eating.

1. I tend to:

    A. Be vigilant about everything I eat and scrutinize food labels.
    B. Eliminate entire food groups. For example, fat or carbs.
    C. Knowingly overeat.
    D. Eat secretively
    E. Crave fresh, homade, natural foods.

2. I often:

   A. Classify food as "good" or "bad".
   B. Engage in strict food rituals.
   C. Feel unable to stop eating.
   D. Purchase large amounts of food at one time.
   E. Purchase fruits and vegetable from the local farmer's market or a CSA farm.

3. Usually, I:

   A. Make food choices based on weight-loss rather than on health.
   B. Accept nothing less than perfection.
   C. Experience irresistible food cravings.
   D. Purge after overeating.
   E. Eat only when I'm actually hungry.

4. I have been known to:

   A. Eat everything I want to before beginning a diet, then I quickly lose resolve once on the diet.
   B. Restrict food intake, even when my body is signaling for food.
   C. Complain about carrying extra weight.
   D. Over-exercise after an unhealthy eating binge.
   E. Exercise moderately on most days.

5. I am:

   A. A yo-yo dieter who experiences constant fluctuation in body weight.
   B. Considered slim.
   C. Aware that I eat more than the average person.
   D. Aware of bloating, gas, GI problems, headaches, thin, dry hair, and brittle nails.
   E. At a healthy weight for my frame, and maintain my weight within a few pounds.

6. I am accustomed to:

    A. Trying every new fad diet that becomes available.
    B. Having a slow metabolism.
    C. Eating very quickly.
    D. Exercising excessively, vomiting, and/or using laxatives or diet pills to prevent weight gain.
    E. Making food choices that positively affect my health.

7. I notice:

    A. That I cut back my food consumption to an unhealthy level.
    B. I experience physical consequences from not eating enough or missing meals. For example: headache, dizziness, loss of concentration, irregular menstrual cycle.
    C. That I often experience weight gain.
    D. That I experience unusual swelling around the jaws.
    E. I usually eat at the same time each day.

8. I know:

    A. I have very strong will-power and have become adept at ignoring what my body needs when it is tired, hungry, aching or sore, because I am determined to be in perfect shape.
    B. I don't have as much energy as I'd like to because I don't eat enough or I over-exercise.
    C. My high blood pressure, fatigue, high cholesterol, diabetes, and/or trouble breathing is a result of my food choices and weight gain.
    D. I lash out at my body when I fail to stick to the severe restrictions I place on my eating.
    E. I have more energy than most people my age.

9. I also know:

   A. Every trick in the book about dieting, calories, and weight-loss.
   B. I can be a bit "obsessive" about my physical appearance.
   C. When I am full, I continue to eat anyway.
   D. I'll have a good day if I get on the scales and weigh less than yesterday.
   E. I look younger than my chronological age.

10. I really believe:

   A. If I find the right diet, I can reach my desired weight.
   B. I'll be more popular and desirable and achieve more if I lose weight.
   C. I am self-conscious, even ashamed about my weight.
   D. One of my greatest fears is to become fat.
   E. Eating well is the secret to health and longevity.

11. Frequently I:

   A. Ignore my body's nutritional needs in order to achieve the weight I want.
   B. Feel fat even though other people tell me I am not overweight.
   C. Feel awkward in social situations because I am overweight.
   D. Experience intense mood swings.
   E. Experience a sense of well-being.

12. I often:

   A. Feel guilty about the least dietary "transgression".
   B. Have difficulty accepting the shape of my own body, and dream of having plastic surgery.
   C. Feel ashamed about how much I eat.
   D. Feel overwhelmed by stress and anxiety.
   E. Feel a strong connection to my spiritual practice.

13. I realize:

   A. That I check other people's bodies and compare myself.
   B. My moods are often based on my eating behavior that day.
   C. I eat small amounts of food in public, but large amounts when I'm alone.
   D. I am very critical of myself in a negative way.
   E. I rarely become sick or catch the latest "bug" going around, and have few if any health concerns.

14. It's true that I:

   A. Often check myself in mirrors.
   B. Often feel disgusted with my body.
   C. Feel others judge me because of my weight.
   D. Base my self-worth on the numbers on the scale.
   E. Try to live harmony with my body and with nature.

Total up how many A's, B's, C's, D's and E's you have.

# of A _____ # of B _____ # of C _____ # of D _____ # of E

The category in which you have the highest total is your eating style.

   A. ***The Perpetual Dieter*** People in this pattern are ever searching for the "magic" diet. They try every new fad diet that comes into vogue. Often these "yo-yo" dieters experience slowed metabolism. In this pattern, the eater knows a litany of facts about food, calories, and dieting tricks, but experiences a disconnection when it comes to nutritional needs. This person is so caught up in the perpetual diet that they fail to experience any joy in eating. A person with this eating style experiences a disconnect from their body in terms of hunger and eating, but also in other mind, body, spirit aspects, such as need for sleep, rest, and recreation. This person tends to over-assert will-power against eating and against themselves in other aspects of their lives. When will-power inevitably falters, guilt prevails. This person may often check themselves in the mirror, or compare their body to that of others.

B. **The Chronic Under-eater** Individuals who experience this eating pattern can be obsessive about eating. They severely restrict their eating, and may even eliminate entire food groups: fats, carbs, and sweets. These people tend to be perfectionists. They may seem vain, but are really insecure about their appearance. Usually these people experience poor body image, and may even think they are fat even when others repeatedly tell them this is not the case. This person my experience low energy due to under-eating, and/or over-exercising, and, at an extreme, may experience frequent headaches, slowed metabolism, or even cessation of menstruation. This person often bases their moods on their eating behavior or the numbers on the scale.

C. **The Over-indulger** This person is typically over-weight. Often they are embarrassed by their weight and by the amount and type of food they eat. A person of this eating style tends to eat very quickly without chewing food well. They feel unable to control their over-eating and battle seemingly intense food cravings. People with this pattern of eating "beat themselves up" for their lack of self-control. They may experience weight-related health issues such as insulin resistance or diabetes, high blood pressure, high cholesterol or difficulty with physical activity. These individuals feel uncomfortable in social situations, believing others are judging them as harshly as they judge themselves.

D. **The Extreme Eater** A person of this eating style tends to binge and purge, but there is a range of extremes. Purging can take the form of over-exercising, use of laxatives, or vomiting. This eater may use diet pills or weight-loss drinks, or go on extreme fasts and cleanses. This person has unrealistic anxiety over becoming fat. He/she assesses self-worth based on the numbers on the scale. They can be harshly self-critical, and have low self-image. Physically this eater will experience the ill-health effects of deteriorating yellowing teeth, yellow eye whites, swelling around the jaws, GI distress, chronic headaches, sallow dry skin, and thin brittle hair and nails. Emotionally, this eater battles anxiety and depression.

E. ***The Enlightened Eater*** The enlightened eater is someone in tune to the rhythms of their body. This person prefers fresh, whole, natural, local and in-season foods. Not only have they cultivated a taste for freshly prepared foods, but they notice how vibrant this makes them feel. They are in tune with their body and notice how eating fast food or junk food affects them physically, mentally, and spiritually. This person has a balanced approach to eating. They eat when they are hungry, and enjoy food as they are eating it. Often they enjoy shopping farmer's markets, participating in a CSA farm, or the process of growing, picking, preparing and eating meals themselves. They are aware of where the food they eat comes from. Physically, they tend to look younger, more trim, and have more energy than other people their own age. They have a high ability to focus and concentrate, and let their body tell them when and what to eat. They get sick less often than other people, and rarely have chronic health concerns. This eater is not at war with food, eating, or their body, but instead they live in harmony with these.

"Knowing others is wisdom, knowing yourself is enlightenment." ~Lao Tzu

Focus for Today: Become aware that the way we eat and treat our bodies is key to making skillful changes. Unproductive eating styles can be changed with awareness and with practice. You don't have to be held hostage by habits that are not working and are not beneficial to you.

Journal: If any of these eating styles are familiar to you, then note it. Awareness is the cornerstone to change.

Recipe of the Day:

Veggie Pot Pie

(Serves 4)

*Organic veggies are preferable
2 carrots, diced
1 small onion, diced
4-5 cloves garlic, chopped
2 potatoes, peeled and cubed into ¼" cubes
½ cup peas or edamame
½ cup corn
2 stalks celery, diced
5 asparagus spears (woody ends removed), cut into ½" pieces
½ tsp thyme
3 Tbsp extra-virgin olive oil
2 ½ cups veggie broth
2 Tbsp flour
Sea salt
Pepper

Sautee vegetables in olive oil until softened. Salt and pepper to taste. Add thyme. Add flour, and mix into veggies. Add broth, stirring until thickened. Pour into pie pan or rectangular Pyrex dish. Top with crust recipe below.

Crust:
1 cup whole wheat pastry flour
¼ cup ground flaxseed
4 Tbsp butter (softened)
Pinch of sea salt
5 tbsp cold water
½ tsp rosemary, crushed into small bits

Mix together dry ingredients. Add butter and mix by hand until mixture looks grainy. Add water. Roll out with rolling pin. Lay dough over veggies. Once the dough tops the pie, use a fork to make several punctures in the crust.

Bake at 350 degrees until crust is slightly brown, 30-40 minutes.

Daily Food Journal

Date:_____   Intention for the day:_____   Weight:_____

Water: *X off one water for every 8 oz. of water that you drink. This includes lemon waters. During a cleanse you should have at least 3 lemon waters daily.*

| YOGI PLATE → | ¼ Protein | ¼ Whole Grains | ½ Veggies |

| Rate your hunger, mood, energy and after meal satisfaction |
| 1=Low   2=Average   3=High |

Time	Meal/ Snack	Food/ Beverage	Hungry?	Mood?	Energy?	Satisfied?
	Breakfast					
	Snack					
	Lunch					
	Snack					
	Dinner					
	Snack					

At the end of the day, reflect on how many servings you had of the following foods/beverages:

Vegetables (Unlimited)	
Whole Grains (Women 1 -3)	
Fruit (Aim for 2)	
Protein (Aim for 3 or more)	

Did I Avoid?	Yes	No	How Much?
Alcohol			
Soft Drinks			
White Sugar			
Artificial Sweeteners			
Processed Food			
Fast Food			

Alert! Use Meat Sparingly

Consume meat no more than 3 times a week!

List your observations and insights for the day. These include successes and behaviors that need attention:

_____
_____
_____
_____
_____

Day 7: *Samskaras*—Self-sabotaging Eating Patterns

"You become that which you think you are. Or, it is not that you become it, but the idea gets very deeply rooted." ~Osho

Samskara, directly translated from Sanskrit, means "deep impression" or "groove" which is set in the unconscious mind. *Samskaras* are patterns and habits which have become so ingrained, we're often not even aware of them. When I think of the word *samskara*, I think of a record album, with the needle stuck in the groove of the record, playing the same thing over and over again. This happens in our lives as well. We often get stuck in unhelpful and unhealthful patterns when it comes to eating and food. So many people believe they are doing all the right things with diet and exercise, and they are scratching their heads because they are still overweight and lacking vitality. During our lifetime, most of us develop our own dietary patterns, grooves or *samskaras.* Oftentimes, people have fallen into patterns or *samskaras* which sabotage their ability to lose weight and feel their best. The following are the six most common eating *samskaras.*

Meal skipping/waiting until you are "starving" to eat: One *samskara,* which people mistakenly think will help them loose weight, is skipping meals or waiting to eat until they are starving. If you have waited to this point, the blood sugar level in your body has crashed! You have already thrown your body completely off balance, and the body is always seeking to return to balance. At this point, your body needs an instant energy boost, so to rebalance itself, it sends out powerful craving signals for foods which provide quick energy. Examples would be simple carbohydrates like crackers, chips, and sugary treats. Eating these sends your blood sugar level skyrocketing, and once again the body needs to rebalance itself. Insulin is released to contend with the surge of sugars found in the simple carbs you have inhaled. It is insulin's job lower blood sugar levels in the blood stream to prevent damage to the organs and tissues, but it is also insulin's job to store the excess sugars in the blood as fat! The constant blood sugar swings up and down lead to insulin resistance, increased fat storage, and slowed metabolism. The body adapts to these swings of intense hunger and carb overloads by slowing the metabolism and storing sugars as fat in anticipation of the next round of meal skipping which it perceives as starvation!

Waiting too long to eat also wreaks havoc on the body. It causes it to go into starvation mode, holding on to each and every calorie, because it doesn't know when or if the next meal is coming. Compounded with that, hunger levels are dramatically increased to protect you from starvation. This causes you to take in an excess amount of calories in the next meal, and then store the excess as fat, just like squirrels store up nuts for the winter! I've had this happen myself when I've been out running errands and missed a meal. I later find myself ravenously hungry, and I end up eating twice or three times the number of calories I would normally eat at a meal. I've heard people say, "I starved myself for a week and gained 2 pounds, I just don't get it!" Starving yourself never works in your favor for weight-loss. Eating the right foods at regular intervals keeps the hunger hormones at bay and allows the body and metabolism to function optimally.

Eating by the clock: Another self-sabotaging *samskara* is eating by the clock. There are many people who eat this way. Instead of listening to their bodies, they watch the clock, letting the clock tell them whether it is appropriate to eat or not. They may not be the least bit hungry, but they eat because it is 6 pm; or they may be weak with hunger, but it is only 5 pm, and they resign themselves to wait out the extra hour! The body knows what it needs and when. The clock is in no way connected to the body. On some days we use more energy than others and need to eat more, or sooner. Other days, we may not have an appetite. As a population, we have become disconnected from our bodies. We need clocks to tell us that we're supposed to be hungry, and we ignore the body's own internal hunger signals: fatigue, lightheadedness, growling stomach, acidity or burning sensations. These signals are warning us that the body is coming out of balance, and we need food to rebalance our energy, hormones, and blood sugar. The body is running out of fuel. We wouldn't let our car run out of fuel, or let the clock dictate when we could put gas in our car! Why then does it make sense that we let the clock tell us when we can refuel ourselves? When we learn to listen to the body and honor what it needs, when it needs it, that's when we come into optimal balance, physically and mentally.

Eating for reasons other than hunger: Eating when we're not hungry is just as problematic! We are so disconnected from our bodies as a culture that we find ourselves eating, not because we are hungry, but because of the Taco Bell commercial we just saw on TV. Or maybe we are eating because the "Moose Track" ice cream just happens to be in the freezer. Sometimes we eat to keep ourselves awake, other times we eat so we can get to sleep, and there are times we eat because we are bored. We may eat because we are stressed or depressed. We are eating and eating, but the one thing we're not is physically hungry! The body didn't ask for these calories. What is it going to do with all of them? The answer is to store them. If a friend comes by your house with a car load of groceries and gives it to you, you can't use it all right away. What do you do? You store it in the freezer, the pantry and the refrigerator! You store it up for when you need it in the future. The body thinks just like you do, *"I can't use this now, but it's a shame to let it go to waste, I'll just store it up!"* The body doesn't have a deep freeze. That extra food goes right to your waist, hips and thighs! If it runs out of room there, it goes on to the back, the back of the arms, the neck and the chin. It will store as much as you give it! The more you store, the longer it takes to use it all up! This is a *samskara* that 60% of American adults have fallen into.

Yo-Yo dieting: Yo-yo dieting is another trap many Americans fall into. People who exhibit this pattern of eating experience considerable weight fluctuations up and down. They tend to try every new diet that comes onto the market, but are unable to stick to these extreme plans permanently, so the weight is quickly regained. Many yo-yo dieters diet during the week and "blow it" on the weekends! These kinds of dieters often take one step forward and two steps back, wreaking havoc on their body and their metabolism. Like the tortoise, slow but steady wins the race. "All or nothing" eating is a dangerous road to travel. The body never knows when it will be starved or gorged, and becomes confused and out of balance. Almost everyone I've met with this eating pattern is overweight. Consistency is everything when it comes to Enlightened Eating.

The endless cycle of food cravings: Food cravings are a *samskara* all of their own. They often take on a life all of their own. Sometimes they are utterly irresistible! According to the ancient healing science of Ayurveda, cravings themselves are a warning sign that an imbalance exists, and they are your body's attempt at bringing itself back into balance. Originally cravings worked as they were intended to for the mind-body system. Before the advent of processed and artificial foods, human cravings were for the specific natural whole-food their bodies needed. We have confused the mind-body system by throwing unnatural laboratory-created foods into the mix. Instead of craving cheese, we find ourselves craving Cheetoes or Cheese-its! Instead of craving orange juice, we crave orange soda. Instead of craving fruits, we crave tutti fruit ice cream! The result is that our bodies never get what they really need and never come back into a state of balance. We continue to hunger, and continue to crave. It becomes a vicious cycle. We become trapped in the pattern of cravings, and eventually the result of imbalance is disease.

When our bodies are getting what they need, the cravings are always satisfied. Excessive or non-stop cravings are a sign of a serious life-style or dietary imbalance. For instance, the most common craving is that of sweets. Sweet cravings can result from low energy reserves, and low-*prana* or life-force, which often arises from excessive exercise, over-work, too little sleep, excessive anxiety or worry, or being too driven in one's ambitions. Very often, sweet cravings come from the lack of "sweetness" in one's way of life. Perhaps you are in a pattern of putting yourself last, or putting up with a job you hate, over-scheduling yourself, a bickering and stressful family life, or a loveless marriage. Perhaps you are too hard on yourself. The lack of "sweetness" in your life can send you seeking sweetness from your pantry and refrigerator. Sweet cravings signal a need for more sweetness, and can actually be eradicated by allowing more "sweetness" to naturally flow into your life by practicing self-compassion and self-care. Give yourself the "sweetness" you deserve. Be sweet to yourself in as many ways as you can and watch the sweet cravings dissolve. Begin to consider new ways of bringing sweetness into your life without the cookies, cakes and candies. If you find that you frequently crave sweets, see if you can satisfy that craving in your life rather than in your mouth. In times when sweet taste is truly what your body is seeking, make sure this sweetness comes from fresh juicy fruits the way nature intended. Satisfying sweet cravings with sugary treats will throw the body out of balance and you will observe new cravings begin to arise as the body seeks to bring itself back into balance. Indulging in sugary snacks often sends people craving something salty!

Craving salt is the second most common craving. This is really a craving for calm. Salt is a mild natural sedative. Salt cravings arise in moments of chaos, nervousness or stress. Craving salty foods can be a result of excessive movement, chaos, work or worry. Salt is an earth mineral which brings about the sense of groundedness which is often missing in our hectic lives. If you find that salt is your downfall, then you are really seeking to relax, calm down and feel more grounded. Why not give your body that which it really desires? Give your mind, body and spirit the calm it truly needs and deserves, instead of pacifying it with salty chips and crackers. If you work to bring more calm into your day, you will notice the salt cravings disappear.

If you find you are craving spicy foods, chocolate, hot peppers, or garlic what you are craving is really energy or stimulation. Spicy foods are natural stimulants. Often people lack energy because they aren't eating foods which contain life-force energy. Processed foods, fast foods, and junk foods actually are depleting to your energy stores and will leave you feeling sluggish. These foods weigh down the metabolism. When energy is low it is because the metabolism is slow. Aromatic, pungent and hot spices rev the metabolism and energy, but only temporarily. Consistently eating natural whole foods keeps the metabolism running at its optimum, and it keeps energy vibrant and steady throughout the day. Too little sleep, over-work, over-exercise, over-stressing and too much caffeine can deplete your energy stores causing your body to seek stimulation. Perhaps it is time to make lifestyle changes in order to maintain energy rather than relying on food as a stimulant. Lifestyle changes are powerful in changing our cycle of cravings.

Comfort foods are called comfort foods for a reason. I think of macaroni and cheese, mashed potatoes, potato salad, and fettuccini Alfredo as quintessential comfort foods. These foods are heavy and weigh down the mind-body system. They are difficult to digest, and dull the senses. Sometimes whether we realize it or not that is exactly what we are seeking. Feeling comfortable is something akin to lounging on a hammock on a warm sunny day. When we are comfortable we feel relaxed and lethargic. When we experience the discomfort of stress and tension, we may seek that sense of comfort and dulling effects from food. It is important to give yourself the comfort your mind, body and spirit are really seeking in life instead of temporarily placating it with food.

When you are not getting enough fluids in your diet, this imbalance can trigger food cravings too. After all, fresh whole foods are 60-80% water. Our bodies tend to crave sweet things in particular because fruits are naturally juicy and naturally sweet. Fresh water is also naturally sweet in taste. At one point in our evolution, the only sweet things we had to satisfy a sweet craving were fresh fruits and naturally sweet fresh water, so this craving served us well and helped rehydrate the body. Now however, sweet cravings send us seeking many things other than fruit. Many of my students have found that by simply having a drink of water, their craving is alleviated. As it turns out when they become conscious of staying hydrated and getting enough fluids, they notice cravings of all kinds diminish. What they were really hungering for was hydration!

Once your body becomes habituated to solving or satisfying its needs for sweetness, calming, energy, and comfort through foods, this becomes a *samskara*. Food becomes a drug rather than a source of nourishment. Cravings can be a difficult pattern to break. However, I know firsthand it can be done. My students are often awed that after the first few weeks of enlightened eating, they notice their cravings are gone. They begin to notice they naturally have more energy, and have calmer, steadier moods without relying on foods. It is very freeing to no longer be a victim of cravings. It is here when they realize cravings are not the norm. When the mind-body system is in balance, we are in control of what we eat instead of food being in control of us.

Once you realize that cravings are simply the result of the mind-body system seeking to bring itself into balance, you have profound awareness. In this awareness, you now have a choice. Foods may be a cheap fix, but they never work permanently. They only last until the next craving arises. We need to become aware of why the craving is arising. Most people are surprised that cravings are not just about food, but what is going on in our life and how we are treating ourselves. Eating the foods our bodies were designed to eat rather than man-made substitutes, helps us return to a state of balance. When we eat in balance, our bodies, minds and spirits come into balance, and the craving cycle is broken. It is here when the craving *samskara* loses its potency.

Convenience food: Probably the most dangerous *samskara* Americans have fallen into is convenience food. The body doesn't get any energy from these foods because this is not the right fuel. It's actually an energy "robber" from the body, because it comes into the body devoid of any life-force energy. However, it takes energy to digest, to process the toxins it contains, and to store. Imagine putting the wrong type of fuel in your car. Let's say you put diet cola in your gas tank. Will your car run at its optimum? Will it even run at all? By putting the wrong fuel into our bodies, we have no energy to exercise, to move; even to do the most ordinary things. People can't figure out why they are so tired. Are they just getting older, or is it what they are putting in to their bodies? It could also be what they are *not* putting into their body that is causing fatigue. When we don't eat life-force containing foods, our own lif-force becomes depleted. When the body becomes sluggish, the mind and spirit are sluggish too.

My 13 year old daughter biked to the local market. She used her own money to purchase a bag of "buffalo wing" flavored pretzels. I didn't say a word. She ate most of the bag. After about half an hour, she began to say she wasn't feeling well. Her head hurt, her stomach didn't feel right, and she felt achy and tired. I read the ingredients on the bag and concluded she hadn't fallen ill, but she was suffering the effect of a virtual chemistry set full of additives, colors, flavors and preservatives.

Samskaras are powerful and difficult to change. The first step in changing them is awareness. Most people stay stuck in these grooves all their lives, never becoming conscious of them, leaving them unable to choose a different course of action. Take notice of your eating patterns throughout the day, throughout the week. Do you recognize any of these common tendencies in yourself? The longer we have held on to these habits, the more difficult they are to break. But we do have the power to change patterns in our lives that are unproductive. Change is our choice. We are not helpless. We must set strong intentions to change. We may find ourselves falling back into the groove again, just like a scratched record or CD repeating the same sound byte over and over. When we find ourselves back in the *samskara*, we must take conscious action to leap out of the groove. I know I have thumped the CD player or jumped up and down to get the CD out of the scratched groove, and move on with the song. We too must take conscious action in our lives, and in our eating. These patterns are actually neuropathways created in the brain. We can create new neuropathways and new patterns. With practice, by repetition, the old *samskaras* lose their strength, and the new neuropathways take over. The old ones become like an unused road, over-grown and eventually impassable. New and better eating habits can be formed! They are life changing! I know, because I've done it! These 40 days are about creating new *samskaras* or "grooves" and strengthening them until the old ones have diminished.

Focus for Today: We all get stuck in continuous cycles and deep patterns in life and in our ways of eating. It is important to be aware that these patterns exist, so we can begin the work it takes to reset and change them.

Journal: Note any patterns or *samskaras* which are familiar to you, knowing that awareness is where the journey begins.

Recipe of the Day:

Crustless Tomato-Basil Tart

(Serves 4-6)

4-5 "meaty" tomatoes, sliced into circles and halved
Hand-full of fresh basil leaves, torn into small pieces
2 large garlic cloves, minced
3 organic eggs
1 cup organic half and half
2 oz grated cheddar cheese
Sea salt and pepper to taste

Layer tomatoes, basil and garlic in ceramic pie dish. Whisk together the eggs, half and half, sea salt and pepper. Pour mixture over tomatoes. Top with cheddar cheese. Bake at 375 degrees for 45 minutes.

Daily Food Journal

Date:_____   Intention for the day:_____   Weight:_____

Water: ☐☐☐☐☐☐☐   *X off one water for every 8 oz. of water that you drink. This includes lemon waters. During a cleanse you should have at least 3 lemon waters daily.*

YOGI PLATE ➡   ¼ Protein ➡
¼ Whole Grains ➡   ½ Veggies

	Rate your hunger, mood, energy		
	and after meal satisfaction		
1=Low	*2=Average*		*3=High*

Time	Meal/ Snack	Food/ Beverage	Hungry?	Mood?	Energy?	Satisfied?
	Breakfast					
	Snack					
	Lunch					
	Snack					
	Dinner					
	Snack					

At the end of the day, reflect on how many servings you had of the following foods/beverages:

Vegetables (Unlimited)	
Whole Grains (Women 1 -3)	
Fruit (Aim for 2)	
Protein (Aim for 3 or more)	

Did I Avoid?	Yes	No	How Much?
Alcohol			
Soft Drinks			
White Sugar			
Artificial Sweeteners			
Processed Food			
Fast Food			

> **Alert! Use Meat Sparingly**
>
> Consume meat no more than 3 times a week!

List your observations and insights for the day. These include successes and behaviors that need attention:

_____
_____
_____
_____
_____

Day 8: Exercise *Samskaras*

"You can't punish yourself into change. You can't whip yourself into shape. But you can love yourself into well-being." ~Susan Skye

We've all been taught that exercise is essential to maintaining weight and health. However, people fall into patterns or tendencies with their exercise regimen, and end up sabotaging their efforts to lose weight, increase energy, and improve health and youthful vitality. Believe it or not, certain exercise patterns can actually be obstacles to achieving the very thing you are working towards!

Excessive/overly strenuous exercise: Excessive or overly strenuous exercise is the most common exercise pattern which sabotages weight, energy, health and youthful vitality. While moderate exercise helps move toxins out of the body, overly strenuous exercise creates toxins. Over-exercising is very aging to the body. According to Ayurveda, intense exercise is said to create *ama* or toxins which accelerate the aging process. Arduous exercisers are not physically different from laborers in the past who toiled from sun-up to sun-down burdened by back-breaking work. They actually aged faster physically, and died younger, than those who paced themselves and worked moderately. I notice how aged marathon runners, tri-athletes or "Iron Man" competitors look. They have a strained look on their faces, deep creases in their skin, and hunched backs. They gray prematurely. I know so many who have had to have knees and hips replaced at surprisingly young ages. I've wondered about people who run excessively: what is it that they are running from? I have a friend whose husband had trained for an Iron Man triathlon. In a year's time his appearance had aged so much that I didn't even recognize him!

People have been led to believe that exercise promotes weight-loss, and if a little is good, more must be better! However, this is simply not the case. Excessive or strenuous exercise stresses the body. Inducing physical stress on the body causes a response similar to psychological stress. The body goes into "fight or flight" mode, and cortisol levels rise. Cortisol is a stress hormone which increases appetite and promotes fat storage. Many people who have spent years exercising strenuously cannot understand why they never seem to lose weight. It is not until they reduce exercise to moderate levels, that the body comes out of "fight or flight" mode and weight-loss occurs. I have heard numerous anecdotes in which people lost 15-30 pounds once they began to exercise in moderation. Recently, a friend of mine posted a photo of herself and her group of fellow marathon runners. Although these women were running at least 2 hours a day in training, each one of them had 15-20 pounds to lose. Although these ladies seemingly enjoy running, clearly all the running has not been a catalyst for weight-loss. In fact, perhaps it has had the opposite effect!

So how do you know if you are exercising excessively or too strenuously? Your exercise regimen should not leave you feeling exhausted, depleted, or devoid of energy for the rest of the day. You should not come away feeling "beat-up" or as if you've just been "hit by a bus!" It is not necessary for your exercise regime to exceed 1 hour a day! After exercising, you should still have time and energy left for other things in life!

Surprisingly to most, healthy weight is 80% eating and only about 20% exercise. It helps to think of exercise more as a way to stay firm, trim and toned in your physique, to keep your bones and muscles strong and to improve cardiovascular health. It takes more than exercising to lose or even maintain weight if you are not eating the foods human beings were designed to eat! Many people mistakenly believe that if only they exercise hard enough and long enough, they can eat whatever they want. This is a huge misconception and there are numerous studies that prove it! We will cover this topic more in Day 18: Enhancing the Metabolism. I do think it is important to tone and strengthen the body, and I have been exercising since I was 16. However, pounding yourself at the gym is never going bring about the optimal you.

Cycle of over-eating, followed by punishing exercise: Another self-sabotaging pattern I've observed is people overeating or eating badly and then trying to "undo" the damage through excessive exercise. Somehow people have come to believe that extra time on the treadmill will negate the all-you-can-eat buffet, or that extra brownie or huge slice of cake! It's almost as if they are physically punishing themselves for their dietary sins, exercising to the point of exhaustion. This is a weight-loss defeating pattern or *samskara*. Excessive exercise saps energy or *prana* (life-force energy, chi, qui; Yoga refers to this energy as *prana*). If all your vital energy is used up on intensive exercise regimes which are motivated by the guilt from a dietary mis-step, you have little energy left for digestion, metabolism, detoxification, healing, the immune system, and anti-aging. You also have little energy left for family, friends and the joy of life! Instead, the body stores up all the energy it can by storing the food you eat as fat, bolstering itself for the next all-out assault it will receive in the form of punishing exercise.

Punishing yourself with exercise places your mind, body and spirit at odds with one another. This is disharmony! A basic principle of Yoga and Ayurveda is *ahimsa* which translates as "doing no harm" or non-violence. This non-harming concept applies to all beings, including you! I've heard people talk about "whipping" themselves into shape or going for a "punishing" run. We've all heard the notion of "no pain, no gain." This is self-inflicted violence! Not only is this way of life unnecessary, but it is actually self-defeating. Yoga seeks to "yoke" or "unite" the mind-body-spirit system by creating harmony among them. Pitting them against each other only sets you up for injury or disease as implied by the word "dis—ease".

Overly intensive exercise creates extreme hunger, because vital nutrients and electrolytes have been depleted from the body. This is followed by over-eating as the body responds to the imbalance, followed by guilt, which results in more punishing exercise regimes, and the cycle goes on. You can't outsmart the body! It is as if the mind and body are at war! The body begins to prepare itself for the next exercise "attack", signaling hunger and storing fat. Weight-loss doesn't happen, and people are wondering how they can work out so hard and so long, with no results to show for it, so they work out even harder! This cycle is futile, like a dog chasing its tail.

I have a runner friend who went for a really long run and was so hungry when she got back, she gobbled down a king-sized bag of M&Ms as fast as she could. This didn't put the needed nutrients back into her body, so she continued to crave things all day. She ate handfuls of this and that, never really satisfying her ravenous hunger, because she wasn't putting in what her depleted body really needed. She felt really guilty for eating so badly and so much, so she was out again at the crack of dawn the next morning to do it all over again caught in the snares of a *samskara*.

Lack of or inconsistent exercise: Just as detrimental to achieving optimal weight, health, energy and vitality is not exercising, or exercising inconsistently or sporadically. The body is designed to move. Movement brings increased blood flow into the muscles and joints and spine, helping them and you to remain healthy, supple, strong and flexible. Exercise works the muscle of the heart, and increases lung capacity. It builds stronger muscles which burn more fuel in the form of calories. Exercise increases bone density, providing protection from osteoporosis. It is the movement of the body which moves lymph through the lymphatic system. Movement helps move waste out of the digestive system. Exercise enables us to eliminate toxins through the skin in the form of sweat. If the body doesn't move enough, *ama* or toxins accumulate in the fat cells. Inevitably the fat cells increase in size as they store more toxins. Research has determined that the bodies of regular moderate exercisers are physically comparable to people 10 years younger.

Find some form of moderate exercise and stick with it the rest of your life. Personally, I am partial to Yoga and walking, but finding something you like and can stick with is a key to health, vitality, and weight management. If you are exercising and wondering why it isn't working for you, perhaps you will recognize yourself in one of these exercise *samskaras*.

"The body has to be loved-you have to be a great friend." ~Osho

"Healing cannot begin until you first make friends with the body." ~Elise Cantrell

Focus for Today: Begin to be aware that it is possible to fall into unhealthy and unproductive patterns of exercise. Identify any of these patterns you notice you have fallen into.

Journal: How are you treating your body? Are you beating it up? Trying to "whip" it into submission, or into shape? What message are you sending it? Are you exercising so much that you have no energy left for enjoying other things in your life? Do you feel depleted? Are you exercising so little that you lack energy and feel sluggish? Are you sending your body love and acceptance, or rejection? Remember your body "hears" every message you send it!

Recipe of the Day:

The Chocolate Monkey Smoothie

(Serves 1)

1 heaping Tbsp organic peanut butter
1 ripe banana
2 heaping Tbsp cocoa powder
4 oz organic milk
1 Tbsp Agave nectar (or to taste, less or more)
Ice cubes (optional for summer months, or recipe can be heated for winter months by using warm or boiled milk)

Blend together above ingredients until smooth. Enjoy!

Daily Food Journal

Date:_____ Intention for the day:_____ Weight:_____

Water: ⬜⬜⬜⬛⬛⬛⬛⬛ *X off one water for every 8 oz. of water that you drink. This includes lemon waters. During a cleanse you should have at least 3 lemon waters daily.*

YOGI PLATE ➡

¼ Protein
½ Veggies
¼ Whole Grains

Rate your hunger, mood, energy
and after meal satisfaction
1=Low   2=Average   3=High

Time	Meal/ Snack	Food/ Beverage	Hungry?	Mood?	Energy?	Satisfied?
	Breakfast					
	Snack					
	Lunch					
	Snack					
	Dinner					
	Snack					

At the end of the day, reflect on how many
servings you had of the following foods/beverages:

Vegetables (Unlimited)	
Whole Grains (Women 1 -3)	
Fruit (Aim for 2)	
Protein (Aim for 3 or more)	

Did I Avoid?	Yes	No	How Much?
Alcohol			
Soft Drinks			
White Sugar			
Artificial Sweeteners			
Processed Food			
Fast Food			

Alert! Use Meat Sparingly
Consume meat no more than 3 times a week!

List your observations and insights for the day. These include successes and behaviors that need attention:

_____
_____
_____
_____
_____

Day 9: Can Yoga Help Me Lose Weight?

Many people have never considered practicing Yoga because they feel they need a more vigorous form of exercise to help them lose weight. What most people don't understand or appreciate is that the practice of Yoga can have powerful weight-loss effects. Studies show that people who practice Yoga regularly weigh, on average, 15 pounds less than non-Yoga practitioners. I believe Yoga has long been overlooked as an effective weight-loss practice. This is because many of the reasons why it works are not obvious at first glance.

The most apparent reason Yoga helps with weight loss is that it is a physical practice which builds long lean muscle, burns calories and tones the body. Many people think of Yoga as "just stretching". However, studies prove that stretching actually burns calories! Out of the estimated 250,000 poses, many are quite challenging and effectively raise the heart rate, working the cardiovascular system even as much as running. Also, many Yoga poses build muscle strength as the body is held in various positions in resistance to gravity. Many Yoga poses are powerful muscle and strength builders. Increasing muscle mass is shown to increase metabolism.

There are also deeper, less obvious reasons why Yoga promotes weight loss. Regular Yoga practice re-balances the endocrine system, which is a key player in weight loss and weight gain. Specific postures target the adrenal, thyroid, pineal and pituitary glands. The pituitary gland regulates and balances all the other glands. The adrenal, thyroid and pineal glands play vital roles in regulating the hormones of metabolism, energy, and hunger. A physical Yoga practice also keeps blood sugar levels in check, along with the accompanying weight gain. Yoga is particularly helpful for women in peri-menopause and menopause battling the "middle-age spread". It helps regulate the hormonal swings up and down, by stimulating the endocrine system to re-balance female sex hormones with each practice. Yoga not only lessens the severity of menopausal symptoms, but also keeps body weight in check.

Another reason Yoga may promote weight loss is that it stimulates the body's own detoxification process. It is known that the body stores toxins in the fat cells. The more toxins that are stored within each cell, the larger that cell becomes. As each fat cell grows, the body expands with it, along with the number on the scales. Toxins are also said to weigh down the metabolism making it sluggish. Yoga postures were designed to move toxins through the lymphatic system, allowing them to be flushed from the body. There are specific postures which stimulate the kidneys and liver, two key organs involved in the body's detoxification process. Other postures stimulate digestion and elimination, the body's first line of defense against toxins. Yoga also promotes sweating, in which toxins are eliminated from the body through the pores. In these ways, Yoga helps the body expel and eliminate toxins, preventing them from being stored in the fat cells, and thus precluding weight gain associated with toxins building up in those cells. With regular practice, toxins already stored in the fat cells will be released and eliminated from the body, resulting in weight loss as well.

Yoga also prevents weight gain by reducing the effects of stress. Yoga is proven to lower blood pressure, heart rate, and stress levels, leaving the practitioner feeling calm, relaxed and with an overall sense of well-being. A Boston University School of Medicine study included in the Journal of Alternative and Complementary Medicine, (Nov. 2010) concluded that practicing Yoga three times a week reduced anxiety remarkably more than walking the same amount of time three times a week. It was noted among the Yoga students that they showed elevated levels of the calming neuro-chemical GABA, whereas the walkers did not show an increased level. Elevated levels of the stress hormone cortisol are well known to stimulate appetite and trigger fat storage particularly in the abdominal area, causing weight gain. Yoga calms stress and releases tension from the muscles and joints and relaxes the mind. Yoga counters what has been termed as the "fight or flight" effect and reduces cortisol levels. Yoga takes us out of our sympathetic nervous system and into the parasympathetic nervous system, promoting relaxation. A regular Yoga practice keeps stress levels and those weight gain hormones associated with stress at bay.

Another less obvious reason Yoga practice helps with weight loss is that it teaches the practitioner to listen to their body. When one learns to listen to the body in Yoga practice, one learns to listen to the body off the Yoga mat as well. It becomes easier to discern whether you are actually hungry, or if you may only be bored or stressed. You become more aware of when you are feeling "full", knowing when to stop eating. You also begin to distinguish what your body is actually craving. You realize that you're not really craving Cheetoes, but cheese instead, perhaps because your body needs the calcium and protein. You begin to listen to the body and not only to your tongue. You get in tune to how your body feels after eating certain foods. You notice which foods energize and revitalize the body, and which foods make you feel tired, cranky, sleepy, or just blah! Once you get in tune with your hunger, your cravings, and with how you feel when you eat certain foods, your eating changes, consciously and unconsciously. You begin to crave clean, nourishing, healthful foods, because you notice how much better they make your body feel. You notice your own energy, stamina, and vitality is directly related to what you put in your body.

A great example of this body awareness comes through a personal story of mine. I had been eating a clean diet for quite some time, when one day (being a southerner) I found myself craving a chili dog. I went and got the chili dog I was craving, and enjoyed every bite . . . until, that is, about 15 minutes later. For the rest of the day I felt tired, lethargic, and just plain yucky. I have never craved a chili dog since! I think many people eat like this all the time, and don't connect their lack of energy, achiness, and overall lethargy to their diet, because they have forgotten what it feels like to truly feel good!

Lastly, I believe Yoga practice decreases the appetite. I personally notice that for at least an hour or two immediately following my Yoga practice, I have no appetite. I have spoken with other Yoga practitioners who experience the same thing. I also notice I have an increased appetite on days when I am unable to practice Yoga. This leads me to suspect that Yoga has both immediate and long term effects on the appetite suppressing hormones. I have no scientific proof of this, but I have come to believe through my own experience and through the anecdotal experience of other yogis, that Yoga does suppress the appetite. This is exactly what diet pills are designed to do, but Yoga does this naturally, without drugs. Yoga practice is a safe and healthy way to naturally achieve ideal weight.

11 reasons Yoga helps with weight loss and weight maintenance:

1. Strengthening Yoga builds lean muscle which burns significantly more calories than fat. One pound of muscle burns 30-50 calories a day vs. the 2-3 calories burned a day by 1 pound of fat.
2. You burn additional calories and fat during and immediately after Yoga practice.
3. Yoga practice includes focus on breathing and breath work or *pranayama,* increasing oxygen levels. Oxygen fuels the "fire" or *agni* of the metabolism according to Ayurveda.
4. Yoga calms stress, lowering the fight or flight response which triggers the hunger hormone cortisol.
5. Specific poses stimulate thyroid and pituitary glands which govern metabolism. Yoga also helps balance many additional hormones in the body.
6. Yoga lowers insulin levels by keeping blood sugar balanced. Insulin stimulates weight gain.
7. Yoga stimulates digestion and elimination.
8. Yoga stimulates the detoxification process. Toxins weigh down the metabolism as well as become stored in the fat cells.
9. Yoga teaches you to listen to your body. You begin to cue into signs of hunger and fullness. You become aware of how eating certain foods makes you feel.
10. Yoga helps the body to balance the hormones. Yoga is great for mid-life or premenopausal weight gain.
11. Yoga curbs the appetite possibly by stimulating the release of appetite suppressing hormones.

Yoga postures, *mudras*, and *bandhas* for weight-loss, metabolism, detoxification and digestion:

Eating within 1-2 hours before or after Yoga practice is contraindicated.

1. **Setu bandha or bridge pose:** Lay on the floor with knees bent. Lift hips off of the floor by pressing into soles of the feet. Weight is on shoulders and feet. Head rests comfortably on the floor. There should be no weight on the neck. Chest

lifts towards chin creating a gentle squeeze in the throat area. Lift, hold and lower three times. This stimulates the thyroid.

2. *Sarvangasana or shoulder stand:* This pose should not be done by persons with neck injuries. This pose compresses and stimulates the thyroid. This pose is best learned under the tutelage of a professional Yoga instructor. The body weight should remain only on the shoulders, not the head or neck. The palms support the mid-back. The chin should be tucked into the chest, which compresses and stimulates the thyroid. The hips, knees and ankles are stacked over the shoulders, and the legs squeeze together. This pose engages an upward lifting energy in which the entire body is lifting up and away from the shoulders towards the ceiling, even as the shoulders are rooting down into the ground.

3. *Halasana or plow pose:* This pose should not be done by persons with neck injuries, and is most safely learned under the supervision of a professional Yoga instructor. This pose also stimulates the thyroid. From shoulder stand position, the legs are lowered over the head, and released to the floor behind the head. The palms press into the floor or the fingers interlace behind the back. If the feet do not reach the floor, it is best to place the feet on a wall behind you, or bend the knees. In this pose there is no weight on the head or neck, only on the shoulders.

4. *Rabbit:* This pose stimulates the thyroid, pineal, pituitary, glands involved in metabolism and regulation of hormones. This pose should not be done by persons with neck injuries and should be learned under direction of a professional Yoga instructor. Seated with sit-bones on heels, one folds forward placing the crown of the head on the floor, and the forehead touching the knees. The hands reach back and hold on to the heels. The sit-bones are then lifted up off of the heels. Most of the body weight remains on the shins. Only about 10% of the weight should be on the crown of the head. The chin should be tucked firmly into the chest.

5. *Body shaking:* While standing, shake the entire body, as if vibrating, for several minutes. This alone will promote weight-loss if practiced 15 minutes a day.

6. *Revolved triangle:* This pose increases digestive fire, metabolism, and targets belly fat. In a standing position, step one foot back approximately a leg-width apart from the front foot. The toes of the front foot point directly forward, and the back foot is at a forty-five degree angle. The hips are squared directly forward facing the front foot. Bending at the hip crease, the opposite hand from the leg that is forward is placed on a block or on the floor on the inside or outside of the front foot. The hand can also be placed on the shin or foot of that leg. Twisting the chest towards the same side as the front leg, the other hand sweeps up and open, rotating the spine. Equal weight is in both feet. The spine lengthens from the tail-bone to the crown of the head, and the front knee remains soft. The gaze is down at the big toe of the front foot, or up at the thumb of the top hand. Repeat on the other side.

7. *One knee wind-relieving pose:* While reclining on the back, one leg is extended. Bend the other knee in towards the underarm, bringing the thigh along the side of the ribcage. Interlace fingers below the knee cap and gently squeeze knee in towards ribs. Both feet are flexed, and both shoulder blades are planted into the floor.

8. *Reverse child's pose:* While reclining on the back, hug both knees into the chest, interlacing the fingers just below the knees. Tuck your chin into your chest and lift your forehead to your knees. Hold. Breathe deeply through the nose. Work up to holding for 1 minute.

9. *Jalandhara bandha:* This pose is a chin lock which stimulates the thyroid gland. Tuck chin firmly into chest, feeling a stretch along the back of the neck. This lock can be done with an internal or an external breath retention. Take a half-swallow to feel the epiglottis lock in place in the throat, making it impossible for breath to escape in or out. Hold until there is a strong urge to breathe. First release the lock, then return to normal

breathing. To increase energy, use along with an internal breath retention. Do not retain breath if pregnant, if experiencing glaucoma, or if prone to migraines or high blood pressure.

10. **Agni mudra:** A hand *mudra*, or Yoga pose for the hands, which is said to promote weight loss, increase the metabolism or digestive fire, and burn excess fat. Fold ring finger of each hand to base of thumb. Press finger with thumb at second phalange. Hold the other fingers straight with purpose and intention. This *mudra* should be practiced in a seated position on an empty stomach only. It should be practiced a minimum of 5 minutes up to 15 minutes. *Agni mudra* builds heat, decreases *kapha* (the water and earth elements contained within the body, which when out of balance can promote weight accumulation), prevents and controls weight gain, and is also said to lower cholesterol. However, *agni mudra* can increase stomach acidity and cause indigestion as a side effect. If this pose causes excess stomach acidity for you, it is best not to include it in your practice. Hand *mudras* have more powerful effects than yoga poses.

Pranayama (yogic breathing) for weight-loss, metabolism and digestion:

(Caution: *Pranayama* should be learned from a professional yoga instructor trained in these techniques. When preformed incorrectly, there can be undesired effects and consequences.)

1. **Kaphalabhati:** Caution: may cause lightheadedness. Always practice seated on the ground. Avoid when pregnant, and if challenged by glaucoma, heart and lung conditions, pace makers, emphysema, recent surgery, migraines or high blood pressure. *Kaphalabhati* literally means "skull polishing". Practicing this breath brings about clarity of mind, illumination, awakening and energizing. It oxygenates the blood and stokes *agni*. **How to:** *Kaphalabhati* is practiced with emphasis on the exhalation. A sharp, crisp burst of air is released through the nose as if trying to blow out a candle through the nostrils. Allow the inhalation to happen involuntarily

and naturally. Place the attention only on the exhalation; trust the inhalation to come automatically. (Do not force or strain on the exhalation, but keep it crisp and short using an abdominal contraction.)

2. ***Bhastrika:*** "Bellows breath" -A Yoga breath which increases the inner fire or metabolism like bellows fan a flame. It is contraindicated for sinus irritation, digestive disorders, heart or lung conditions, pregnancy, menstruation, high blood pressure, migraines or glaucoma. This technique may also cause lightheadedness and should be practiced seated on the ground. **How to:** In this breath equal attention is given to the inhalation and the exhalation. With a strong inhalation, the rib-cage expands and the ribs widen apart. With a strong exhalation, the ribcage contracts inward. The breaths are steady and even, never forced or strained. Attention remains focused on the strong expansion and contraction of the ribs. Repeat for 20 breaths. **Advanced variation:** Arm movement is employed with the breath. Option 1- Arms with fists extend forward at shoulder height upon inhalation, and retract back to the sides of the ribcage upon exhalation. Option 2- Arms with fists extend upward overhead upon inhalation, and retract back to the sides of the ribcage upon exhalation.

3. ***Ujjai:*** "Darth Vader" breath, performed by constricting the back of throat while breathing in and out of the nostrils. An audible "ocean-like" sound should be heard upon inhalation and exhalation.

4. ***Uddiyana bandha kriya:*** This is not only a *pranayama* or breath technique, but also a *kriya* or cleansing practice. It involves a series of external breath retentions along with the engagement of a diaphragmatic "lock" or *bandha.* It is said to increase *agni,* the internal digestive fire, thereby increasing the metabolic capacity as well as the ability to "burn away" toxins. It is important to practice this technique on an empty stomach. It is contraindicated for recent surgery, pregnancy, menstruation, high blood pressure, heart conditions, stroke or glaucoma. **How to:** Stand with feet hip width apart, knees bent. Place palms on thighs, and lock the elbows keeping arms straight. The

back is flat, at a 45-degree angle. Inhale deeply, and then exhale completely. Use abdominal muscles to push out any breath remaining in the lungs. Hold the breath out. Then, draw the diaphragm in and up into the abdominal cavity locking it in a concave position. Hold this position and the breath until there is a strong urge to breathe. First release the diaphragmatic lock, and then inhale. Repeat the process several times for 3 to 10 rounds.

5. *Agni sara kriya:* This is a more powerful expression of uddiyana bandha kriya. This technique carries the same precautions and contraindications. In this technique, while the exhalation is being held out, the diaphragm locks and releases. As it releases, the abdominal muscles are pressed out rounding the belly forward. Then the abdomen and diaphragm are contracted back in and up. The abdomen will move through cycles of becoming concave then convex, until there is a strong urge to breathe. After the lock is released for the final time, breathe in. Return to normal breathing for several breaths, and then repeat for 3-10 rounds. This is a powerful practice which is said to purify toxins, and rev agni. It intensifies body heat, the metabolism, and the immune system.

Yoga practice to enhance the metabolism:

You will find a sequence of poses below designed to flow one into the other in a single session. This sequence is designed to promote increased metabolism.

1. *Agni Mudra:* Thumb holds down ring finger to base of thumb on both hands. The other fingers fully extend.
2. *Ujjai pranayama:* "Darth Vader" breath, constricting the back of throat while breathing in and out of the nostrils.
3. *Bhastrika:* "Bellows" breath. This breath is reputed to increase *agni* the fire of the metabolism, and is said to have a decisive impact on health and vitality. This breath should be learned and practiced via a professional Yoga instructor.

4. **Spinal rocking:** On back, knees bent, feet a comfortable distance away from sitz bones. This stimulates the central nervous system.

5. **Windshield wiper-knees:** Move knees side to side. Hold knees on right side, twist. Hold on left side, twist. Stimulates the intestines for elimination.

6. **Bridge pose:** Reclining on the back, bend the knees and place the feet a comfortable distance away from the sitz bones. Lift hips off of the floor by pressing into soles of the feet. Weight is on shoulders and feet. Head rests comfortably on the floor. There should be no weight on the neck. Chest lifts towards chin creating a gentle squeeze in the throat area. Lift, hold and lower three times. Stimulates thyroid.

7. **Windshield wiper:** Knees move side to side in a slow windshield wiper motion. Hold knees on right side, twist. Hold on left side, twist. Stimulates the intestines for elimination.

8. **Down dog or puppy dog:** With hands and feet on the floor move into an inverted letter "v". Hands are shoulder width apart. Feet are hip width apart. Fingers are spread wide. Weight is on the full hand, not just the wrist. Heels are sinking down towards the floor. Sit-bones are pressing up towards the ceiling. Puppy dog is a modification in which this pose is done on the knees instead of the feet.

9. **Ragdoll:** A standing forward fold, in which feet are hip width apart, knees are slightly bent, and hands clasp opposite elbows. The head hangs freely.

10. **Mountain pose:** Standing, as if a mountain. Feet are hip width apart firmly rooted into the earth, arms spread out to sides as if the slopes of a mountain, and crown of head reaches upwards as if the peak of a mountain.

11. **Forward fold:** Bend the upper body forward at the hip crease, hands or fingertips touch or reach towards the floor. Knees are slightly bent.

12. **Down dog:** Walk hands back to feet and roll up to standing.

13. **Chair pose:** Standing with feet hip width apart, sit back as if there is an invisible chair behind you. Palms are in prayer position at heart center. Twist to the right, bringing the left elbow or hand to the outside of the right knee. Rest by coming into a standing forward fold. Return to chair, and twist to the left.

14. **Gorilla pose:** Standing with feet hip width apart, fold forward at the hip crease. Allow the knees to remain soft with a slight bend. Place palms under the soles of feet, standing on the hands. Modify by holding calves or ankles. Hold for several breaths.

15. **Triangle pose:** Standing at the front of the Yoga mat, step one foot back one leg length apart from the front foot. Toes of front foot pointing forward and back foot perpendicular to front. The front toe and heel should line up with the arch of the back foot. Shift weight into the back hip, reach forward with the front hand and then float it down to the shin of the front leg. Raise the other hand up towards the ceiling. Gaze can be down at the big toe, or up at the raised thumb.

16. **Revolved triangle:** This pose stimulates digestion and elimination, increases internal "fire", and tones abdominals. This pose is said to reduce belly fat. In a standing position, step one foot back approximately a leg-width apart from the front foot. The toes of the front foot point directly forward, and the back foot is at a forty-five degree angle. The hips are squared directly forward facing the front foot. Bending at the hip crease, the opposite hand from the leg that is forward is placed on a block or on the floor on the inside or outside of the front foot. The hand can also be placed on the shin or foot. Twisting the chest towards the same side as the front leg, the other hand sweeps up and open, rotating the spine. Equal weight is in both feet. The spine lengthens from the tail-bone to the crown of the head, and the front knee remains soft. The gaze is down at the big toe of the front foot, or up at the thumb of the top hand. Hold for several breaths.

17. **Eagle pose to eagle fold:** Also stimulates digestion and elimination and internal "fire" and tones abdominals, hips thighs. Standing, wrap the right leg over the left. Toe can touch the floor or a block to aid with balance. Right arm wraps under the left, so that the right elbow cradles the left elbow. Hands come together, either palm to palm or knuckles to knuckles. Elbows lift to shoulder height. While wrapped up begin to sit back as if lowering towards a chair. Hold for several breaths.

18. *Wind relieving poses*:

    A. With one knee: Reclining on back, one leg is extended. Bend the other knee in towards the underarm, thigh along the side of the ribcage. Interlace fingers below the knee cap and gently squeeze knee in towards ribs. Both feet are flexed, and both shoulder blades are planted into the floor.

    B. With two knees: Hug both knees into chest. Tuck chin into chest and lift forehead to knees. Hold. Breathe deeply through the nose. Work up to holding 1 minute.

    These poses relieve lower back pain; help with gas, constipation, and acidity; improve digestion and elimination; stimulate weight-loss especially in the abdominal region; tone abdominals and reduce belly fat.

19. *Shoulder stand:* This pose stimulates thyroid. This pose should not be done by persons with neck injuries. This pose compresses and stimulates the thyroid. This pose is best learned under the tutelage of a professional Yoga instructor. The body weight should remain only on the shoulders, not the head or neck. The palms support the mid-back. The chin should be tucked into the chest, which compresses and stimulates the thyroid. The hips, knees and ankles are stacked over the shoulders, and the legs squeeze together. This pose engages an upward lifting energy in which the entire body is lifting up and away from the shoulders towards the ceiling, even as the shoulders are rooting down into the ground.

20. *Plow pose:* This pose stimulates the thyroid. It should not be attempted by persons with neck injuries, and is most safely learned under the supervision of a professional Yoga instructor. From shoulder stand position, the legs are lowered over the head, and released to the floor behind the head. The palms press into the floor or the fingers interlace behind the back. If the feet do not reach the floor, it is best to place the feet on a wall behind you, or bend the knees. In this pose there is no weight on the head or neck, only on the shoulders.

21. **Fish:** This pose opens throat after it has been compressed in shoulder stand and plow to stimulate the thyroid. This creates a "rinse and soak" action in this gland which regulates metabolism. Reclining on the back, place the hands under the hips, palms facing down. Bend elbows sliding the head onto the crown, exposing the throat. The neck and chest will lift off of the floor. The top of the head, the buttocks, the legs and feet are on the floor. This pose is not for someone with neck issues.

22. **Seated head to knee pose:** Lock chin to chest. Stimulates thyroid.

23. **Rabbit pose:** This pose stimulates the thyroid and releases shoulder and neck tension. Only about 10% of weight is on the crown of the head, 90% is on knees, shin and feet. Contraindications: not for persons with neck issues. Kneeling with sit-bones on heels, fold forward placing the crown of the head on the floor, and the forehead touching the knees. The hands reach back and hold on to the heels. The sit-bones are then lifted up off of the heels. Most of the body weight remains on the shins. Only about 10% of the weight should be on the crown of the head. The chin should be tucked firmly into the chest.

24. **Hero pose:** Kneel with sit-bones on heels, calves tucked under thighs.

25. **Twisted lord of the fishes pose:** This pose stimulates the thyroid as well as digestion. From a seated position, bend one knee in towards the chest and place the sole of that foot on the outside of the thigh of the extended leg. Bring the opposite elbow to the outside of the bent knee, the palm of this hand makes a "stop sign" as you come into a spinal twist. Press the elbow into the knee gently as the head turns to look over the shoulder. The "sitz" bones should root into the mat and the crown of the head should lift towards the ceiling keeping the spine long so that the vertebrae have plenty of space in which to rotate.

26. **Reclining twist:** Lying on the back, reach the arms out to the sides at shoulder level. Draw the knees into the chest, and let them fall to the right. Hold for several breaths, and then, shift the knees to the left and hold.

27. *Savasana:* This pose is also called corpse pose. Lie on the back in a comfortable position, with palms open towards the ceiling, hands resting by the sides. Close the eyes, and allow the feet to fall open and gravity to take over. Bring your attention to your breath.

Focus for Today: Yoga does help you lose weight, and the reasons go well beyond the obvious!

Journal: In what ways do you believe Yoga can help promote optimal weight for you?

Recipe of the Day:

This recipe is a delicious and easy way to enjoy summer's delicious tomatoes.

Roasted Heirloom Tomato-Basil Soup

3 lbs heirloom tomatoes, chopped into large pieces
1 yellow onion, chopped into large pieces
2 carrots, chopped into large sections
½ head of garlic peeled
1 stick organic celery
Extra virgin olive oil
1 large bay leaf
4 cups organic vegetable broth
Handful of fresh basil
Sea salt and pepper

Preheat oven to 450 degrees. Place all vegetables on a roasting pan and drizzle with olive oil, and sprinkle with sea salt and pepper. Roast vegetables in oven about 25 minutes, until caramelized. Remove from oven and place vegetables in large Dutch oven on stove top. Add vegetable broth and bay leaf and simmer for 20 minutes. Add basil last and puree with puree wand or in a food processor. Salt and pepper to taste. Serve and enjoy!

Daily Food Journal

Date:_____ Intention for the day:_____ Weight:_____

Water: [water cup icons] X off one water for every 8 oz. of water that you drink. This includes lemon waters. During a cleanse you should have at least 3 lemon waters daily.

YOGI PLATE ➡ ¼ Protein ➡ [plate diagram] ⬅ ½ Veggies
¼ Whole Grains ➡

| Rate your hunger, mood, energy |
| and after meal satisfaction |
| 1=Low   2=Average   3=High |

Time	Meal/Snack	Food/Beverage	Hungry?	Mood?	Energy?	Satisfied?
	Breakfast					
	Snack					
	Lunch					
	Snack					
	Dinner					
	Snack					

At the end of the day, reflect on how many servings you had of the following foods/beverages:

Vegetables (Unlimited)	
Whole Grains (Women 1 -3)	
Fruit (Aim for 2)	
Protein (Aim for 3 or more)	

Did I Avoid?	Yes	No	How Much?
Alcohol			
Soft Drinks			
White Sugar			
Artificial Sweeteners			
Processed Food			
Fast Food			

| Alert! Use Meat Sparingly |
| Consume meat no more than 3 times a week! |

List your observations and insights for the day. These include successes and behaviors that need attention:
_____
_____
_____
_____
_____

Day 10: Enlightened Eating OUT!

Eating out either for pleasure, for business or for convenience is unavoidable in today's fast-paced world. However, eating out frequently can severely sabotage your efforts towards achieving your ideal health, weight, energy and vitality. Here are some of the biggest pitfalls of eating out:

1. ***Fast Food:*** Fast food actually is "slow food" because it causes us to feel slow, lethargic and sluggish. It causes us to feel this way because it is full of chemical flavors, colors, additives and preservatives, and it has been processed to the point that it no longer contains any nutritional benefits or value. When food causes us to feel sluggish, it is because the metabolism slows, leading to lethargy. This lethargic feeling leads us to be less active. Low activity level is another sure-fire way to gain weight.

    I remember the 1990s fast food mantra "Super-size me!" meaning add an extra large soda and extra-large fries. Well it worked! America is now super-sized! Talk about setting intentions! Currently, 30% of American adults are obese, and another 30% are over-weight. The fast food industry uses every marketing strategy available to get you to order more and to keep you coming back, all in the name of profit. Their arsenal of strategies even includes adding chemical flavor enhancers, as well as chemical appetite enhancers. These are the same kind of tactics used by the tobacco industry. Both industries are largely responsible for America's health crisis. As the fast food industry expands its bank accounts, we expand our waist lines and our health care spending. Enlightened eaters stay away from fast food establishments!

2. **Buffets:** These are a disaster waiting to happen. A buffet in and of itself is deliberately setting you up to overeat. In buffets, low-quality processed food sits under heat lamps for hours on end, with FDA regulation "sneeze guards" in place to supposedly help hold the proliferation of germs at bay. The only life-force these foods contain is the bacteria rapidly multiplying in them! Do not walk, run from buffet restaurants! These shouldn't even enter into the decision process for an "enlightened eater". Ayurveda asserts that overeating is *tamas* creating dullness, heaviness, and lethargy, while also producing toxins in the body due to the inability to process large quantities of food efficiently.

3. **"Diners, Drive-ins and Dives":** Even though some of the food here may be homemade, the foods in these eating establishments are notoriously "greasy", fried, heavy, and come in enormous portions. This is a sure-fire way to sabotage your enlightened eating. I was actually on an episode of this captivating program starring Guy Fieri several years ago. While visiting my hometown and family, I was coaxed into going along with them to a famous local drive-in. Not surprisingly, there was nothing "enlightened" on the menu! I certainly have not made the best eating choices at every moment of my life, but I have become increasingly enlightened by paying the consequences physically for eating foods which did not serve my body! I still remember how awful I felt after finishing that infamous meal!

4. **Chain restaurants:** Chain restaurants may have some better options than fast food restaurants, buffets, and diners, however, bear in mind that the foods they serve are pre-prepared, and stored up or frozen and trucked in to restaurants all over the country and even the world. The result of this is poor quality, lack of nutrients, and little if any life-force energy in the foods. In order for foods to remain edible during the transporting process, preservatives are added.

5. **Let the names of the dishes be your clue!:** "Loaded" baked potato soup really means it is *loaded* with fat and calories. We began the 40 days by talking about the power of intentions. Menu items' names set the intention for the

meal, and for your weight and health. Just look at what happened with the "super size me" intention! Here are some examples: "bottomless tortilla chips", you'll keep eating because they keep coming and they'll go straight to your bottom! "All-you-can-eat soup, salad and bread sticks": one bowl of soup, one breadstick, and one small salad is sufficient for any adult. One should never eat all they possibly can! This sabotages weight, metabolism, and health. I also believe it distorts your sense of how much food is really necessary and OK. "Quesadija Grande": grande means large, and it will make you large too! "Sinful chocolate cake": is sure to send you to confession! "Death by chocolate"—need I say more? These are a few examples, but there are many more. Let the names give you insight into what you order, and into what intentions you are setting for your meal and for how you wish to look and feel.

How to navigate eating out the "enlightened" way:

1. **Go local:** Look for restaurants that serve fresh, local, organic foods. These restaurants receive their food fresh daily, so it still contains valuable life-force energy or *prana*. The food is prepared fresh daily, so you are not eating processed food loaded with preservatives. You dollar is supporting the local economy from the farmer to the restaurant owner, unlike a chain restaurant headquartered in another state.

2. **Choose wisely:** If you must eat at a fast food or chain restaurant, look for the most nutrient-dense option on the menu. McDonalds now has berry smoothies, and oatmeal with walnuts, sweetened with maple syrup. People get caught in the pitfall that they might as well throw in the towel since they are eating out, and order things they'd never normally eat at home. Thankfully due to public demand, there are better options out there than there once were. Also, be sure to not feel obligated to order dessert just because you are eating out.

3. **Plan ahead:** Don't wait until you are famished to choose where you will dine. This is a downward spiral, because our intentions can be de-railed by intense hunger. When we are super hungry, our menu choices are more likely not to be items that honor or serve our body and health. In many cases you can view restaurant menus on-line in advance to determine whether there are enlightened choices. Planning ahead averts disaster!

4. **Ask your body:** Listen to what your body needs, not to your taste buds. Only the tongue can actually taste food, but the entire body benefits or becomes affected by what goes in. Don't allow those few inches of taste buds to override your innate wisdom as to what is best for your body. Let your body make your food choices, not your tongue. Ask your body what it needs today. It will tell you. (And it won't be the "chili-cheese smothered fries")

5. **Use your imagination:** Imagine the basket of dinner rolls on your hips. If you eat all the bread they bring out, that's where you will see it! There is a strategy the restaurants use with these rolls. Bread makes you thirsty, and they are hoping you will order more drinks, which have an enormous mark-up! These rolls are doing neither your hips nor your wallet any favors!

6. **Order water for your drink:** Ask for a lemon, and you will receive the benefits of the lemon water discussed earlier. You will rehydrate your body and save yourself the non-nourishing calories of cocktails or sodas. It may be a good idea in restaurants, to squeeze the lemon into the water and set the rind aside, getting the benefits of the lemon without the sprays on the peel, unless you are certain that the lemon is organic!

7. **Halve your portion:** Most restaurant portions could serve a family of four! Split your meal with someone else and save money while you are saving your weight and health. Or box half to take home immediately before eating. Out of sight, out of mind. If the meal was not an optimal choice, just leave the box on the table when you leave. Remember left-overs quickly lose their nutrients and begin to develop bacteria and toxins, beginning

to decompose within 2 hours. Left-overs and reheated foods are not recommended in Ayurveda. Left-overs have begun to lose their *prana* or life-force energy! Do not eat left-overs over 24 hours old unless they were immediately placed in the freezer.

8. **Survive the airport:** Air travel is a huge challenge to enlightened eaters! You are a virtual prisoner to the food choices available on the plane or in the airport . . . or are you? With a little planning, ingenuity and creativity, you can circumvent the tasteless, lifeless, expensive stuff that is airport food. I have begun packing a meal in my carry on, complete with paper plate, plastic fork, napkin, etc. An example of a meal I might bring is a pouch of tuna, a pouch of Poupon mustard, nuts, organic whole-grain crackers, and a fruit such as strawberries, an apple or orange. I also bring an empty water bottle, so I can fill it with water after going through security. This is not ideal, but it travels well and is a better choice than airport food! It is said that an airplane is drier than the Sahara Desert, so it is critical to stay hydrated. The dry nature of air travel is one of the reasons many people complain of constipation after a flight. Drinking plenty of water helps. I also bring several tea bags (organic teas) and ask for hot water on the plane, rather than soda. For snacks in case I experience long delays, I bring organic tamari roasted almonds, dark organic chocolate, dry roasted edamame, and another fruit such as an apple or clementine.

9. **Car travel:** When you are imprisoned in the car for hours at a time, convenience stores and fast-food restaurants can seem the easiest alternative. However, with a little planning, you can avoid the junk-food, fast-food, processed-food trap. When you are planning to spend time on the road, I suggest bringing bottles of water, flavored carbonated water, and bottles of all-natural or organic teas as refreshing drinks. Bring along a couple of lemon slices to add to your water, and receive the benefits of lemon water. For snacking, bring packets of nuts such as organic tamari almonds, sunflower seeds, Lara Bars, Kind Bars, and easy to eat fruits such as apples or pears.

Fresh carrots are easy to eat while you are driving as well. The main thing is to come prepared when you will be spending time in a car, so you won't resort to foods you will later regret.

10. **Hotels:** When you are staying in a hotel, it is a challenge to stay on track with your eating. Challenging as it is, it is possible to navigate hotels relatively unscathed. Most hotels have a mini fridge in which you can store your own fruit, veggies, and healthful beverages. I even bring my organic lemon slices along for my morning cup of hot lemon water. If worse comes to worse, you can use hot tap water for this, or bring along an electric kettle. Usually hotels have a coffeemaker in the room and this is a great way to heat your water. There is also no reason to use the hotel's coffee if you bring your own organic coffee along. I usually bring several healthy bars for breakfast or snacks. I also like to bring along some nuts and organic fruit to keep on hand.

11. **Party survival:** I suggest offering to bring a dish to pass at the party to "help" the hostess. Then prepare and bring something delicious and healthful. At least you'll know you have something there at the party that you can eat with a clear conscience. This will also open up a discussion with your friends about Enlightened Eating as they "Oooo and Ahh" over your dish. They will discover that eating nourishing foods can taste great too! I recommend that you stick with water and a lemon or lime, sparkling mineral water, or some other healthful beverage. Alcohol lowers your inhibitions at parties, and the snack table will become more and more tempting! Make sure you stand away from the snack table while chatting with friends. I try to not even cast a glance at it. Even better yet, stand and chat in another room. Standing and chatting by the snack table is a sure fire way to fall victim to temptation!

These are a few of my own strategies to navigate eating out and travel in the most enlightened way possible. Although these situations are not easy, there is no reason to completely derail your eating weight and health!

Focus for Today: Eating out, travel or parties do not have to be set-backs in your quest towards your optimal health, weight, and self. Awareness, planning, and making informed choices are key. Being consistent is crucial!

Journal: How can you make better choices when you eat out, party or travel? What have you been doing in the past when dining out, travel and parties may have been sabotaging your goals? What is your new strategy?

Recipe of the Day: Enjoy the enlightened recipe today. It is a terrific option to bring to a party or pot-luck, giving yourself and others a healthy option!

Colorful Quinoa Salad

2 cups organic quinoa
4 cups water
½ red onion, chopped
4 green onions, chopped
1/3 cup slivered almonds
½ cup dried cranberries
Large handful of chopped Italian parsley

The dressing:
Juice of 1 organic lemon
Zest of ½ organic lemon
1 Tbsp Dijon mustard
4 cloves garlic
1 organic apple sliced-to add sweetness
¼ cup expeller pressed canola oil
Sea salt and pepper to taste

Bring the water and quinoa to boil and cook over low heat until water is evaporated. Allow to cool to room temperature. Mix in onions, almonds, "Craisins", and parsley. Put the dressing contents into blender and liquefy. Pour the dressing over quinoa salad and mix thoroughly. Enjoy warm or cold!

Daily Food Journal

Date:_____   Intention for the day:_____   Weight:_____

Water: ⬜⬜⬜⬛⬛⬛⬛⬛   *X off one water for every 8 oz. of water that you drink. This includes lemon waters. During a cleanse you should have at least 3 lemon waters daily.*

YOGI PLATE	←

¼ Protein
½ Veggies
¼ Whole Grains

Rate your hunger, mood, energy and after meal satisfaction

1=Low   2=Average   3=High

Time	Meal/Snack	Food/Beverage	Hungry?	Mood?	Energy?	Satisfied?
	Breakfast					
	Snack					
	Lunch					
	Snack					
	Dinner					
	Snack					

At the end of the day, reflect on how many servings you had of the following foods/beverages:

Vegetables (Unlimited)	
Whole Grains (Women 1 -3)	
Fruit (Aim for 2)	
Protein (Aim for 3 or more)	

Did I Avoid?	Yes	No	How Much?
Alcohol			
Soft Drinks			
White Sugar			
Artificial Sweeteners			
Processed Food			
Fast Food			

Alert! Use Meat Sparingly

Consume meat no more than 3 times a week!

List your observations and insights for the day. These include successes and behaviors that need attention:

_____
_____
_____
_____
_____

Day 11: It's Not How Much You Eat as Much as What You're Eating

"We are living in a world today where lemonade is made from artificial flavors and furniture polish is made from real lemons." ~Alfred E. Newman

We've all at some point tried counting calories, carbs, fat grams or points. With all this counting, why aren't we losing weight? Most people don't realize that it's not how much you eat, as much as what you eat! I know people who are carefully counting each calorie, but they can't lose weight. Often, it is not about the calories, but about the food they are eating and what it contains or lacks. Eating processed foods that lack nutrients causes people to hold on to weight in a couple of ways. First, the body is actually hungry for nutrients, and even though it is getting something resembling food, it continues to hunger for what it really needs. When it receives junk instead, the body goes into starvation mode trying to store each and every calorie, mistakenly believing it is starving. The body slows down the metabolism to hold on to every calorie it can, because it is starved of what it really needs.

Second, people continue to hunger because their bodies haven't received real food or real nourishment! Cravings continue, no matter how much junk food or processed food the body has received, because it is seeking the nutrients contained in real wholesome foods. The body continues with hunger and cravings because it is created to hunger until it gets what it needs, and that only comes from foods it was designed to consume. I believe there are some over-weight and even obese people out there who are actually "starving"! Their bodies are literally nutrient, micronutrient and antioxidant deprived, yet their bodies are inundated with substances that they don't need and cannot use. In addition, these foods overload the body with toxins. Energy and vitality is quickly depleted as the body deals with an overload of toxins and a deficit of nutrients. I see this in people whose diets consist mainly of processed and fast foods. They may not even eat that much calorie-wise, but they can't seem to lose weight.

The obvious solution may seem to be taking a multi-vitamin/multi-mineral supplement. However, the body cannot be tricked! The body knows the difference between laboratory created vitamins and those naturally occurring in fresh, wholesome food. Science is just beginning to discover the micronutrients which whole foods contain and the optimal combination of these as they occur in nature. Vitamin pills do not contain these newly discovered essential nutrients, and large doses of certain vitamins actually block the absorption of other vitamins, minerals, and nutrients. Amazingly it has been found that whole foods actually contain nutrients in the perfect combinations and amounts. The body cannot be deceived. When the body doesn't get all the nutrients it needs to function optimally, it induces more cravings, leaving you constantly hungry, prone to "cave in" and over-eat as it is seeking what it needs. I will repeat this many times through this book: *the body is always seeking to be in balance.* If we don't consciously bring the body into balance, it will take charge on its own. This is what it is programmed to do. We can work with it or against it, but the body cannot be fooled. By simply eating foods which nutritionally satisfy the body's needs, you will be amazed by the decrease in appetite and increase in energy that results.

We have become convinced that a calorie is a calorie. If this were true, 60% of American adults would not be overweight or obese. Technically, a calorie is a calorie, but not to our bodies. For example, six diet sodas a day net 0 calories. But it has been proven that people who drink diet sodas actually weigh quite a bit more than those who do not. People think they are fooling their bodies with diet drinks, but I'll repeat it again, the body cannot be fooled. The "sweet" taste alone can cause weight gain even if no sugar is found. In Ayurveda, excess sweet taste is said to increase bodily tissue and create *Ama* or toxins! Sweet taste regardless of the number of calories it lacks or contains is known in Ayurvedic science to build body mass. It is best to slowly begin to decrease your taste buds' sensitivity to sweetness if you are looking to decrease body mass. It is not about the calories. I did this myself, and over time began to consciously decrease the amount of sweeteners I used a little at a time. Now it takes very little sweetener to satisfy me, and now I am actually repelled by overly sweet foods!

A calorie is not a calorie when it comes to how often you eat. Studies show that if you eat five or six smaller meals, keeping the body fueled and running evenly all day, you'll lose more weight than eating the same number of calories at three larger meals. This makes sense, because your body is receiving a more steady supply of energy throughout the day. You will feel more energized throughout the day as well, maintaining a continuous supply of calories and energy. There will be no crash; no time slumped on the couch. The blood sugar will not plummet, creating the ravenous cravings of a starving lion! Instead the body will maintain a steady supply of insulin and a steady, healthy blood sugar level. Also, eating large meals dampens the digestive fire, or metabolism, as the system becomes overwhelmed. By eating several smaller meals, the digestive fire stays at its optimum and the body doesn't have to hoard calories waiting many hours until the next meal.

A personal experience with the concept of "a calorie really is not a calorie" came during a 10-day stay at Kripalu Center for Yoga and Health. The food there is delicious, fresh, homemade, and 100% organic and Ayurvedic. During my stay, I ate more than usual, often going back for seconds. At the same time, we also did a good bit more sitting than I ordinarily do, taking notes, watching demonstrations, practicing meditation and *pranayama* or breath work. I was shocked when I got home and found that I had lost 2 ½ pounds. It wasn't how much I ate or moved around, it was clearly what I was eating.

A similar story comes from a friend of mine who made a 2-week trip to Mexico. When she came back, she told me she had eaten more than ever, and so had her children. They were incredulous to discover that when they returned home, they had each lost about 5 pounds. She said the only difference from home was that every day they went to the farmer's market and bought everything fresh for preparing that day's meals. Simply by eating fresh foods, their bodies began to shed weight. This made her a believer!

Notice that there is no calorie counting or measuring in the "Enlightened Eating" philosophy. There is no need to "starve "yourself in order to lose weight! There is no need to go hungry at all. Diets that leave you feeling hungry almost always backfire, because your body begins to think it is starving. Since the body is always seeking to be in balance, it increases the hunger and fat storage hormones it releases, in order to protect you from starvation!! For years we've been told all we have to do is limit the calories we take in or burn them off. This tactic simply hasn't worked. When it comes to eating, quality is what really matters. Here is a quote from Jessica H., one of my Enlightened Eating students. *"Wow Elise, now I know it's not about the calories! I lost 5 pounds in the first week and I'm feeling great!"*

Focus for Today: By now you have noticed we are not counting calories. Enlightened Eating isn't about calories and measuring. Quality of food is much more important when it comes to achieving your ideal weight and health.

Journal: Discuss anything you have noticed in your own experience of how eating certain kinds of food can affect weight more so than cutting calories.

Recipe of the Day:

Citrus-Avocado-Almond Salad

Organic baby salad greens
Fresh oranges, peeled and sliced, white pulp removed
Avocado, peeled and cut into slices
Almond slivers
Red onion, thinly sliced
Toss together and drizzle with the dressing below.

The dressing:
(serves 4-5)

½ cup olive oil
½ cup citrus juice (grapefruit, orange, lemon)
3-4 cloves fresh garlic
Piece of peeled ginger (the size of the tip of the thumb)
3 Tbsp Bragg's Aminos
Sea salt to taste
Pepper to taste
Blend the above ingredients in blender.

Daily Food Journal

Date:_____ Intention for the day:_____ Weight:_____

Water: ☐ ☐ ☐ ■ ■ ■ ■ ■ ■ *X off one water for every 8 oz. of water that you drink. This includes lemon waters. During a cleanse you should have at least 3 lemon waters daily.*

		Rate your hunger, mood, energy

YOGI PLATE ➡

¼ Protein ➡
½ Veggies
¼ Whole Grains

Rate your hunger, mood, energy
and after meal satisfaction

1=Low   2=Average   3=High

Time	Meal/Snack	Food/Beverage	Hungry?	Mood?	Energy?	Satisfied?
	Breakfast					
	Snack					
	Lunch					
	Snack					
	Dinner					
	Snack					

At the end of the day, reflect on how many servings you had of the following foods/beverages:

Vegetables (Unlimited)	
Whole Grains (Women 1 -3)	
Fruit (Aim for 2)	
Protein (Aim for 3 or more)	

Did I Avoid?	Yes	No	How Much?
Alcohol			
Soft Drinks			
White Sugar			
Artificial Sweeteners			
Processed Food			
Fast Food			

Alert! Use Meat Sparingly

Consume meat no more than 3 times a week!

List your observations and insights for the day. These include successes and behaviors that need attention:

_____
_____
_____
_____
_____
_____

Day 12: Starting Over

"Let go of perfection,
There are no mistakes,
Only learning.
Accept where you are,
embrace your resistance,
and be open to growth through experience.
Honor your humanity,
and learn from all teachers".
~Anonymous

One day while meditating, I heard these words in my head. *"Perfection is imperfection, and imperfection is perfection."* It was a revelation, a kind of breakthrough for me. These words brought tears streaming down my face. I am a "recovering" perfectionist. I realized that if God had really wanted to create everything including humans "perfect", he could have and already would have done it. It dawned on me that he *has* created perfection. Perfection is *imperfection.* In my imperfection, I am perfect just as I am. We are all already perfection just as we are, and we are not perfect. Therein lies our unique beauty and perfection.

Meditation itself is an exercise in imperfection. The goal of many forms of meditation is to keep the mind focused on the breath or a fixed object such as a candle, flower, picture, mantra or a fixed point in space. Whenever the mind wanders away from this point of focus, and it inevitably will, you simply recognize that it has drifted, and return the mind back to its original focal point. In meditation, again and again, and again, it is necessary to gently direct the mind back to its focus. Eventually, the mind wanders less and less frequently. Eventually focus is trained. Ultimately you are able to stay longer and longer without drifting away, and those moments are pure bliss.

Life as well is an exercise in maintaining focus and confronting inevitable imperfection. However, life also gives us as many chances as we need to start over again and give things another go! Eventually we get it right! Enlightened Eating works the same way. Slip-ups happen. Setbacks can happen on any journey! Slip-ups in which you lapse into your old ways of eating can happen during the 40 days. These old patterns, grooves or *samskaras* may be familiar and comfortable, but you know they haven't worked in your favor. Instead of beating yourself up, it is important to learn from setbacks. *"When Perfection Ends, Beauty Begins." ~Dr. Gopala Aiyar Sundaramoorthy*

My enlightened eating students have had their biggest moments of realization from relapse into eating things they used to eat and noticing how awful they felt afterwards. One student had to sleep almost sitting up after giving into a meal at a local Mexican restaurant because her heart burn was so bad! Another student noticed how badly her joints ached after indulging in processed food. Another student almost became physically ill after ingesting salad greens with a chemical taste on them. One of my students made a few small slip-ups one week during the 40 day process, and was really disappointed that she didn't lose any weight that week. Over Christmas break, I got a bit lax with my own eating, and I began to notice my joints aching, I felt heavy, bloated and stiff, and my energy became sluggish. These setbacks were great teachers. Imperfection is inevitable, but learning from it is certain. Each time we wander away from our ideal way of eating, the opportunity is always there to return to our focus, to return to our intention, and begin a little wiser. To stay on the path, and make change permanent, we must begin again as many times as it takes to get it right.

At the beginning of the 40 Days we discussed the importance of having a "beginner's mind". A beginner's mind is one that is always willing to begin again. It is essential not to become derailed by a dietary mis-step or slip-up along the journey. Look at these moments as a learning opportunity, and an opportunity to practice "beginner's mind" by starting over rather than giving up. Giving up is not an option if you are truly seeking transformation. As long as you are willing to start over, as many times as it takes, you will see results and your intentions will be realized.

The 3-day cleanse is a great way to return back to our focus which is the intention we set when we began Enlightened Eating and eating in alignment with the mind, body and spirit. If you find that you have lost focus on eating in an enlightened way, simply start over, return to the cleanse for 3 days. Doing this is like pressing your own "reset" button and it refocuses you back on your intention. It is ok to start over as many times as it takes to become enlightened! After the 40 days is over, I invite you to start over and repeat the 40 day journey as many times as it takes to stay focused without drifting back into old ways of eating which weren't serving you mind, body and spirit. As a teacher of 40 Days to Enlightened Eating, I repeat the 40 days along with each group I lead. With each group experience, my awareness expands, my trust in the process deepens, my focus sharpens, and my ability to remain engaged in eating the right foods increases.

"Each morning we are born again. What we do today is what matters most." ~Jack Kornfield

*"Have patience with all things, but chiefly patience with yourself. Do not lose courage in considering your imperfections, but instantly set about remedying them; everyday begin the task anew." ~St. Francis de Sales

Focus for Today: Starting over. Return focus on the intentions you set at the beginning of the 40 days. Re-read the intentions written in your journal and refresh yourself with your initial resolve. Perhaps you need to repeat the 3-day cleanse. Do whatever it takes for you to return your focus to the Enlightened Eating plan and to your intentions. Remember "beginner's mind" (see Day 1). Throughout the entire 40 Days we are still beginners. Perhaps you need to start over and begin again!

Journal: Rewrite your intentions. Have they changed? What are you struggling with? In what aspects of the plan do you need to start over?

Recipe of the Day:

Southwestern Black Bean Salad with Creamy Chili-Lime Dressing

(Serves 2)

4 cups salad greens including some bitter greens such as swiss chard, kale, or beet greens
¼ red onion, finely chopped
½ cup organic corn
½ cup organic black beans, rinsed
½ avocado, chopped
1 medium tomato, chopped
1 small cucumber, chopped

For the dressing:

4 oz oil of your choice
Juice of 1 large or 2 small limes
¼ cup Greek yogurt
2 cloves garlic
3 tsp taco seasoning
Sea salt and pepper to taste

Blend together the dressing ingredients until smooth. Drizzle over salad.

Daily Food Journal

Date:_____   Intention for the day:_____   Weight:_____

Water: ☐☐☐☐■■■■   *X off one water for every 8 oz. of water that you drink. This includes lemon waters. During a cleanse you should have at least 3 lemon waters daily.*

YOGI PLATE ➡

¼ Protein ➡
½ Veggies
¼ Whole Grains ➡

Rate your hunger, mood, energy		
and after meal satisfaction		
1=Low	2=Average	3=High

Time	Meal/ Snack	Food/ Beverage	Hungry?	Mood?	Energy?	Satisfied?
	Breakfast					
	Snack					
	Lunch					
	Snack					
	Dinner					
	Snack					

At the end of the day, reflect on how many
servings you had of the following foods/beverages:

Vegetables (Unlimited)	
Whole Grains (Women 1 -3)	
Fruit (Aim for 2)	
Protein (Aim for 3 or more)	

Did I Avoid?	Yes	No	How Much?
Alcohol			
Soft Drinks			
White Sugar			
Artificial Sweeteners			
Processed Food			
Fast Food			

Alert! Use Meat Sparingly
Consume meat no more than 3 times a week!

List your observations and insights for the day. These include successes and behaviors that need attention:

_____
_____
_____
_____
_____

Day 13: The 3 *Gunas* of Eating

"Do not overlook tiny good actions, thinking they are of no benefit. Even tiny drops of water in the end will fill a huge vessel." ~Buddha

According to Ayurveda and Yoga philosophy, three primordial qualities or *gunas* exist in all things in the universe. These qualities are called *rajas*, *tamas* and *sattva*. In all things, one of the three qualities is predominant. *Rajas* is a state of motion, activity, agitation, energy and change. *Tamas* is a state of darkness, heaviness or inertia. *Sattva* is a state of harmony, balance and purity. The best way to imagine these qualities in food is to imagine a banana. In its *rajas* state, the banana is green and ripening, but not ideal for eating. In its *tamas* state, the banana is brown, decomposing, and devoid of life-force; again, not ideal for eating. In its *sattvic* state, the banana is at the peak of ripeness and purity, its life-force is optimal, and it is perfect for eating. One of the three *gunas* is dominant in all foods, and as in the case of the banana, and the quality of foods is ever-changing. The same three *gunas* play a role in our day-to-day eating as well. Although most people eat foods in all three of their varying states, some people eat more foods which are *sattvic* or pure, others eat more foods which are *rajasic* or agitating, and others eat more foods which are *tamas* or heavy, dull and inert. Our own human state of being can be *rajas*, agitated, *sattva*, pure and harmonious, or *tamas*, dull and inert. Our own predominant *guna* or quality of character is directly affected by the underlying qualities or *gunas* of the foods which dominate our diet.

The following is a "3-*Guna*" self-quiz. Check and see which of the three *gunas* is predominant in your eating. This will give you a good idea whether you yourself are in a state of agitation, inertia or harmony. Answer these questions based on the way you ate before you began the 40 Days of Enlightened Eating.

Is my eating *Rajas*, *Tamas*, or *Sattva*?

(Check the one that applies in each row.)

1. I most often eat: _____ homemade food _____ in restaurants _____ reheated prepared, convenience foods.
2. I often eat my fruit and vegetables: _____ fresh _____ dried or canned _____ I don't like fruit or vegetables.
3. I often buy my food at: _____ the local farmer's market _____ the supermarket _____ the convenience store.
4. My diet is: _____ vegetarian _____ some meat _____ heavy meat.
5. I tend to: _____ chew each bite 20 times _____ eat rapidly _____ over-eat.
6. I stop eating at: _____ 70-80% full _____ 100% full _____ 120% or more full.
7. I eat: _____ at regular times each day _____ sporadically or skip meals _____ by "grazing" all day.
8. I order pizza delivery or pick up take-out: _____ rarely _____ once or twice a month _____ weekly.
9. I drink alcohol: _____ rarely or never _____ 1 or 3 drinks/ week _____ daily.
10. I use tobacco: _____ never _____ only when I drink alcohol _____ daily.
11. I use caffeine or stimulants: _____ never _____ few times/week _____ several times daily.
12. My favorite foods are: _____ natural foods _____ fried foods _____ fast foods.
13. I sweeten with: _____ natural sweeteners _____ white sugar _____ artificial sweeteners.
14. I prefer: _____ whole grains _____ white bread, flour, rice _____ Cheetoes, Doritoes, and doughnuts.
15. I enjoy drinking: _____ herbal teas or fruit juices _____ sports drinks _____ diet soda.
16. I exercise: _____ moderately and regularly _____ hardcore _____ sporadically if at all.
17. I practice Yoga: _____ moderately at least 3 times/week _____ hot or power Yoga _____ rarely.

18. I sleep: _____ 7-8 hours/night _____ erratically or too few hours _____ 9 hours or more.
19. I crave: _____ fresh whole foods _____ salty or spicy foods _____ junk food.
20. Usually my food is: _____ organic when possible _____ convenient _____ left-overs.

The first choice in each row is *sattva*, the second is *rajas*, and the third is *tamas*. Total your check marks for each.

Total: _____ *sattva* _____ *rajas* _____ *tamas*

No matter what your score, keep in mind that all three *gunas* exist in unison in everyone and everything. However, a yogic and ayurvedic eating philosophy seeks to cultivate a mostly *sattvic* way of eating.

The *Sattvic* Diet:

The *sattvic* way of eating is the most ideal, purest diet. A *sattvic* diet is said to cultivate the qualities of harmony, balance, lightness, joy and positivity. It promotes functioning at the highest potential in the mind, body and spirit. This diet is said to create optimal health, as it nourishes the entire being. The mind is peaceful and relaxed and functions in a clear and balanced state. A healthy body and peaceful mind pave the way for a deepened spiritual connection where spiritual growth flourishes. Yoga and Ayurveda see a direct relationship between your physical and mental health and thriving spiritually. The true goal of these sister sciences is to cultivate the health and harmony of all three *gunas*. A *sattvic* state of being is actually the state of having the ideal balance between motion and energy, and dullness and lethargy, being neither agitated, nor sluggish. It is in this state of balance where peace and calm are found.

A *sattvic* diet is fresh, juicy, light, and nourishing. It is seasonal, organic, free of processed or artificial foods, chemical-free, fresh, and natural. These foods are filled with nutrients and are said to be burgeoning with life-force or *prana*. *Sattva* in eating is best represented by eating fresh picked tomatoes in summertime, or eating strawberries right off the vine. *Sattvic* foods include whole grains, fruits and vegetables, juices, nuts, seeds, legumes, and dairy products (excluding eggs), and including natural herbs, spices and sweeteners. These foods are ideally prepared fresh, lightly cooked (as opposed to over-cooked or raw), and not eaten as left-overs. Eating this way the majority of the time will impart unparalleled support to the immune system. It will enhance energy, vibrant health, ideal weight, youthfulness and vitality. A *sattvic* diet encourages compassion, emotional balance, contentment, and mental clarity. Moreover, a *sattvic* diet is said to help bring about self-realization, nourish a more virtuous, holy nature, and fertilize the seeds of enlightenment. The proverb "cleanliness is next to godliness" certainly applies here in terms of eating and food. The cleaner the diet is, the purer the mind and spirit. When you are craving *sattvic* foods, you are craving a feeling of lightness and clarity as well as nourishment and steady energy.

The *Rajas* Diet:

Rajas is probably the most common way of eating in modern society. This way of eating only exacerbates over-stimulation, imbalance and agitation. By over-exciting our system with *rajas* foods, the mind experiences chatter, distraction, and difficulty focusing and concentrating. By consuming disproportionate amounts of *rajasic* foods, restlessness, impatience and distractibility are aggravated. Ego and desires of every kind begin to overpower the psyche. Anxiety, excessive talking, thinking, eating, exercising, and a variety of exaggerated urges can arise. In the extreme, this can result in hyperactivity and even lead to an array of addictions. Foods that encourage *rajas* tendencies are greasy, spicy, overly salty, overly sweet, dry, sour or bitter. Caffeine, tobacco, chocolate, hot peppers, garlic and onions (alums), mushrooms, fish, eggs, white flour, white sugar, and anything deep fried is considered *rajas*. Onions, garlic and mushrooms, eggs and fish do have redeeming nutritional value, but are considered *rajas* due to their natural stimulating effects. Over consumption of these foods tends to agitate the mind-body system, and weaken the spiritual connection in deference to the ego. Historically, *Rajas* foods were intentionally fed to Indian armies in order to intensify agitation, flare the temper and increase the nervous energy essential for battle. Although these foods are acceptable in appropriate quantities, limiting the intake of these foods to a modest percentage of the diet is recommended to promote harmony and balance physically, mentally and spiritually. When you crave *rajasic* foods, you are really craving quick energy mentally and/or physically. For example: a college student studying late at night for exams, or someone who is performing some strenuous physical task might be someone who is craving *rajasic* foods.

The *Tamas* Diet:

Tamasic eating is the most potentially harmful of all three *gunas*. *Tamasic* foods are depleting and devoid of life-force or *prana*. They are old, decaying and consume more vital energy to digest and process in the body than they impart. These foods are heavy, impure, contain toxins, and are said to foster complacency, low-energy, darkness, lethargy and inertia. These foods release poisons into the body during the digestive process, and thereby cloud and dim the mind leading to dullness. These foods weigh down the body and slow down its systems, including the metabolism. They not only reduce immunity, but promote disease. These foods can cultivate depression, sloth, grasping, clinging and apathy. *Tamasic* foods include meat, processed foods, fast food, canned foods, left-overs, over-cooked foods, stale or overripe foods, artificial flavors, sweeteners, preservatives, colors, alcohol and other fermented foods. Over-eating is also said to promote a *tamasic* state mind-body and spirit. *Tamasic* foods in excess cultivate a lower animal-like nature in the mind.

Decreasing and/or avoiding these foods can reverse existing health conditions, weight accumulation, and the effects of aging and disease. Furthermore, rapid improvement in energy, mental clarity, and luster of the hair, skin and nails will occur. Over-all life-force will be enhanced. Feelings of heaviness, depression and lethargy diminish. When you are craving *tamasic* foods you are craving a feeling of groundedness and stability. People tend to crave these foods when they are feeling agitated because they impart a sense of weight and heaviness. *Tamasic* foods bring about dulling the senses much like a drug.

It is important to note that the three *gunas* can be used with intention when it comes to eating. For example, on days in which a lot of energy and "fire" is needed you may intentionally eat more warming spices like cinnamon, ginger or peppers. On days in which more focus, concentration and sense of "lightness" are desired, you would want to choose a more *sattvic* diet such as fresh juicy fruits and vegetables. On occasion, *tamasic* foods are used in Ayurveda to bring about a sense of heaviness or inertia. For example, a patient in a manic state may be given red meat to weigh their system down and create a sense of dullness. You might even observe that you intuitively select foods which encourage the state of awareness you wish to have on a given day. It is important to note that saints, sages, and gurus are known to opt for a primarily *sattvic* diet. A *sattvic* diet nourishes a higher level of awareness and lightness of being. It is equally important to note that studies have shown that persons with criminal backgrounds tend to eat primarily *tamasic* diets. Studies have shown that when more *sattvic* meals of fresh fruits and vegetables are served in prisons, violence is significantly reduced.

With these Ayurvedic eating principles in mind, is it not overly difficult to observe a person's behavior, emotional state and physical appearance, and guess their diet or the state of their spiritual condition. For example, people who are very ego driven tend to eat a more *rajasic* diet. People who are slow and sluggish and lack moral and ethical values tend to eat a more *tamasic* diet. People who are calm, harmonious and upbeat in mood and energy tend to eat a more *sattvic* diet. In Yoga and Ayurveda, the mind, body and spirit are intricately interwoven and are codependent on one another in order to thrive. By nurturing the body, we in turn are nurturing the mind and spirit. When one of these begins to heal, the others heal too.

The table below summarizes how to eat in order to cultivate more *Sattva:*

Increase sattvic foods	Reduce rajasic foods	Avoid/eliminate tamasic foods
Fresh organic fruits, vegetables, berries, juices	Fried foods	Fast food, processed food, junk food, convenience food
Whole grains Legumes Spices: ginger, cinnamon, cardamom	Overly salty foods, overly sweet foods	Artificially sweetened, colored, flavored or preserved food, GMO (genetically modified) food
Nuts, seeds	Hot, spicy foods	Canned foods, frozen dinners
Natural sweeteners: honey, stevia, agave, molasses, raw sugar	Caffeine, chocolate, stimulants	Over-cooked, reheated, or leftover foods
Oils: olive or sesame	White flour, white sugar	Meat, particularly red meat
Organic, hormone-free dairy	Fish, eggs	Stale or overripe foods
Herbal teas	Alums: garlic and onions, mushrooms— these are healthy but stimulating foods	Alcohol, fermented foods

Focus for Today: The most important point today is the realization that foods we eat affect the quality of our mental and spiritual health as much they do our physical health. Healing the body heals the mind and soul. Begin to notice connections between what you eat and the mood that follows.

Journal: What category did most of your food choices fall into? Is this a surprise? What can you tweak to improve the health of your mind-body-spirit? Were you aware of the strong connection between what you eat and your mind and spirit? Record any connections you have noticed between foods you eat and moods, emotions and energy.

Recipe of the Day:

Enlightened Squash Casserole

(Serves 4)

2 large summer squash, sliced in circles and quartered
1 medium yellow onion, chopped
½ red bell pepper, cubed
¼ cup fresh chives, chopped
2 cloves garlic, minced
½ cup grated sharp cheddar cheese
½ cup grated parmesan cheese
1 cup non-fat Greek yogurt
2 organic eggs
2 Tbsp olive oil
½ cup organic whole grain cracker crumbs (I use crushed Back to Nature Organic Stone-ground Wheat Crackers)
Sea salt and pepper to taste

Preheat oven to 350 degrees. Sautee the squash, onion, pepper and garlic in olive oil. Sea salt and pepper to taste. Whisk together the yogurt, grated cheese, chives, eggs, add dash of sea salt and pepper. Stir together sautéed vegetables and yogurt mixture in casserole dish. Cover the top with cracker crumbs. Bake in preheated oven for 35 minutes.

Daily Food Journal

Date:_____ Intention for the day:_____ Weight:_____

Water: X off one water for every 8 oz. of water that you drink. This includes lemon waters. During a cleanse you should have at least 3 lemon waters daily.

YOGI PLATE ➡ ¼ Protein — ½ Veggies — ¼ Whole Grains

Rate your hunger, mood, energy
and after meal satisfaction

| | 1=Low | 2=Average | 3=High |

Time	Meal/ Snack	Food/ Beverage	Hungry?	Mood?	Energy?	Satisfied?
	Breakfast					
	Snack					
	Lunch					
	Snack					
	Dinner					
	Snack					

At the end of the day, reflect on how many
servings you had of the following foods/beverages:

Vegetables (Unlimited)	
Whole Grains (Women 1 -3)	
Fruit (Aim for 2)	
Protein (Aim for 3 or more)	

Did I Avoid?	Yes	No	How Much?
Alcohol			
Soft Drinks			
White Sugar			
Artificial Sweeteners			
Processed Food			
Fast Food			

Alert! Use Meat Sparingly

Consume meat no more than 3 times a week!

List your observations and insights for the day. These include successes and behaviors that need attention:

_____
_____
_____
_____
_____

Day 14: What is Your *Dosha*? Determining Your Ayurvedic Constitutional Type

"Know thyself." ~Nitzsche

Human beings are not exactly alike. A primary principle behind the science of Ayurveda is the fact that we are each composed of a unique nature or constitution. In each individual, there are varying proportions of three different "primordial natures" which come together uniquely to compose who we are and how we are. It is the degree to which each of these forces exists within us, that our individual characteristics are manifested. Our constitution or "biological humor" falls into three main categories. These categories classify the human physical, mental and emotional characteristics into three types or *doshas: vata, pitta,* and *kapha.* Although, varying degrees of all three *doshas* exist in everyone, often the characteristics of one *dosha* will be predominant. This is said to be the person's makeup or constitution and defines the individual's innate nature as far as physical characteristics as well as personality traits. This constitution is unchangeable, and exists from conception. There is no need to judge or try to change someone's constitution, since this is impossible to do. There is no right or wrong constitution, and one constitution is not better than another. They are just different. Simply put, your *dosha* is your own blueprint for your physical, mental and emotional self. It is, however, possible for the *doshas* to develop imbalance. Since everyone has varying amounts of all three *doshas,* any of the three *doshas* can become imbalanced in someone. However, it is easiest for a person's predominant *dosha*(s) to become imbalanced. The characteristics of each of the three *doshas* will be described and explained in detail after you have taken the *dosha* test below.

The following Ayurvedic constitutional self-quiz was developed by Dr. David Frawley, director of the American Institute of Vedic Studies. Dr. Frawley is the foremost Ayurvedic expert in the western world. This quiz can be found in his book Ayurvedic Healing page 31-34. There are many versions of Ayurvedic *dosha* quizzes, but I think this one is very thorough. Simply circle the best answer in each row. If you feel that two answers in the same row are completely equal, then it is fine to circle both of the answers. At the end, total up the number of circled answers in each column. The column in which you have the highest total is your dominant *dosha*. It is not uncommon for a person to be *bi-doshic*, having two *doshas* with about the same number of answers. Being *tri-doshic*, balanced in all three categories is somewhat more rare, but is also a possibility.

AYURVEDIC CONSTITUTIONAL TEST

BODILY STRUCTURE AND APPEARANCE

	Vata	Pitta	Kapha
FRAME	Tall or short, thin; poorly developed physique	Medium; moderately developed physique	Stout, stocky, short, big; well developed physique
WEIGHT	Low, hard to hold weight, prominent veins and bones	Moderate, good muscles	Heavy, tends towards obesity
COMPLEXION	Dull, brown, darkish	Red, ruddy, flushed, glowing	White, pale
SKIN TEXTURE AND TEMPERATURE	Thin, dry, cold, rough, cracked, prominent veins	Warm, moist, pink, with moles, freckles, acne	Thick, white, moist, cold, soft, smooth
HAIR	Scanty, coarse, dry, brown, slightly wavy	Moderate, fine, soft, early gray or bald	Abundant, oily, thick, very wavy, lustrous
HEAD	Small, thin, long, unsteady	Moderate	Large, stocky, steady
FOREHEAD	Small, wrinkled	Moderate, with folds	Large, broad
FACE	Thin, small, long, wrinkled, dusky, dull	Moderate, ruddy, sharp contours	Large, round, fat, white or pale, soft contours
NECK	Thin, long	Medium	Large, thick

	Vata	Pitta	Kapha
EYEBROWS	Small, thin, unsteady	Moderate, fine	Thick, bushy, many hairs
EYELASHES	Small, dry, firm	Small, thin, fine	Large, thick, oily, firm
EYES	Small, dry, thin, brown, dull, unsteady	Medium, thin, red (inflamed easily), green, piercing	Wide, prominent, thick, oily, white, attractive
NOSE	Thin, small, long, dry, crooked	Medium	Thick, big, firm, oily
LIPS	Thin, small, darkish, dry, unsteady	Medium, soft, red	Thick, large, oily, smooth, firm
TEETH AND GUMS	Thin, dry, small, rough, crooked, receding gums	Medium, soft, pink, gums bleed easily	Large, thick, soft, pink, oily
SHOULDERS	Thin, small, flat, hunched	Medium	Broad, thick, firm, oily
CHEST	Thin, small, narrow, poorly developed	Medium	Broad, large, well or overly developed
ARMS	Thin, overly small or long, poorly developed	Medium	Large, thick, round, well developed
HANDS	Small, thin, dry, cold, rough, fissured, unsteady	Medium, warm, pink	Large, thick, oily, cool, firm
THIGHS	Thin, narrow	Medium	Well-developed, round, fat
LEGS	Thin, excessively long or short, prominent knees	Medium	Large, stocky
CALVES	Small, hard, tight	Loose, soft	Shapely, firm
FEET	Small, thin, long, dry, rough, fissured, unsteady	Medium, soft, pink	Large, thick, hard, firm
JOINTS	Small, thin, dry, unsteady, cracking	Medium, soft, loose	Large, thick, well built
NAILS	Small, thin, dry, rough, fissured, cracked, darkish	Medium, soft, pink	Large, thick, smooth, white, firm, oily

WASTE MATERIALS / METABOLISM

	Vata	Pitta	Kapha
URINE	Scanty, difficult, colorless	Profuse, yellow, red, burning	Moderate, whitish, milky
FECES	Scanty, dry, hard, difficult or painful, gas, constipation	Abundant, loose, yellowish, diarrhea, with burning sensation	Moderate, solid, sometimes pale in color, mucus in stool
SWEAT / BODY ODOR	Scanty, no smell	Profuse, hot, strong smell	Moderate, cold, pleasant smell
APPETITE	Variable, erratic	Strong, sharp	Constant, low
TASTE PREFERENCES	Prefers sweet, sour or salty food, cooked with oil and spices	Prefers sweet, bitter or astringent food, raw, lightly cooked, no spices	Prefers pungent, bitter or astringent food, cooked with spices but not oil
CIRCULATION	Poor, variable, erratic	Good, warm	Good, warm, slow, steady

GENERAL CHARACTERISTICS

	Vata	Pitta	Kapha
ACTIVITY	Quick, fast, unsteady, erratic, hyperactive	Medium, motivated, purposeful, goal seeking	Slow, steady, stately
STRENGTH / ENDURANCE	Low, poor endurance, starts and stops quickly	Medium, intolerant of heat	Strong, good endurance, but slow in starting
SEXUAL NATURE	Variable, erratic, deviant, strong desire but low energy, few children	Moderate, passionate, quarrelsome, dominating	Low but constant sexual desire, good sexual energy, devoted, many children
SENSITIVITY	Fear of cold, wind, sensitive to dryness	Fear of heat, dislike of sun, fire	Fear of cold, damp, likes wind and sun
RESISTANCE TO DISEASE	Poor, variable, weak immune system	Medium, prone to infection	Good, prone to congestive disorders

	Vata	Pitta	Kapha
DISEASE TENDENCY	Nervous system diseases, pain, arthritis, mental disorder	Fevers, infections, inflammatory diseases	Respiratory system diseases, mucus, edema
REACTION TO MEDICATIONS	Quick, low dosage needed, unexpected side effects or nervous reactions	Medium, average dosage	Slow, high dosage required, effects slow to manifest
PULSE	Thready, rapid, superficial, irregular, weak / like a snake	Wiry, bounding, moderate / like a frog	Deep, slow, steady, deep, rolling, slippery / like a swan

MENTAL FACTORS AND EXPRESSION

	Vata	Pitta	Kapha
VOICE	Low, weak, hoarse	High pitch, sharp, moderate, good tone	Pleasant, deep, good tone
SPEECH	Quick, inconsistent, erratic, talkative	Moderate, argumentative, convincing	Slow, definite, not talkative
MENTAL NATURE	Quick, adaptable, indecisive	Intelligent, penetrating, critical	Slow, steady, dull
MEMORY	Poor, notices things easily but easily forgets	Sharp, clear	Slow to take notice but will not forget
FINANCES	Earns and spends quickly, erratically	Spends on specific goals, causes or projects	Holds on to what one earns, particularly property
EMOTIONAL TENDENCIES	Fearful, anxious, nervous	Angry, irritable, contentious	Calm, content, attached, sentimental
NEUROTIC TENDENCIES	Hysteria, trembling, anxiety attacks	Extreme temper, rage, tantrums	Depression, unresponsiveness, sorrow
FAITH	Erratic, changeable, rebel	Determined, fanatic, leader	Constant, loyal, conservative

	Vata	Pitta	Kapha
SLEEP	Light, tends towards insomnia	Moderate, may wake up but will fall asleep again	Heavy, difficulty in waking up
DREAMS	Flying, moving, restless, nightmares	Colorful, passionate, conflict	Romantic, sentimental, watery, few dreams
HABITS	Likes speed, traveling, parks, plays, jokes, stories, trivia, artistic activities, dancing	Likes competitive sports, debates, politics, hunting, research	Likes water, sailing, flowers, cosmetics, business ventures, cooking

Totals _____ *Vata* _____ *Pitta* _____ *Kapha*

The column with the most items circled indicates your dominant *dosha*. The more dominant a *dosha* is, meaning the higher the total in one column, and the larger the discrepancy there is between the dominant *dosha* and the other *doshas*, the more attributes of that *dosha* a person will have. Remember some people are a near balance of two *doshas*, and a few people are balanced between all three. Ayurveda recognizes seven different constitutional types: *vata, pitta, kapha, vata-pitta, vata-kapha, pitta-kapha*, and *vata-pitta-kapha*(V-P-K) or *tri-doshic*.

Vata: The *vata dosha* takes on the characteristics of air and ether elements or wind. It is dry, light, cold, active, erratic and inconsistent. *Vata* persons can be likened to birds due to their small, light bones and flighty nature. They are similar to the gazelle or antelope, moving lightly and swiftly. They often, but not always, appear physically lean and lithe.

A person having a predominantly *vata* constitution will appear thin, flat chested, have small eyes, long arms, dry frizzy hair, dry skin, and thin weak nails. *Vatas* are "small boned", appearing more fragile than the other *doshas*. Their posture tends to hunch slightly at the shoulders with the head protruding forward. Due to dryness, the skin is prone to premature aging. The dryness/air characteristic of their nature promotes cracking noises in the joints and makes this *dosha* is more prone to arthritis. There is also a tendency to have excessive intestinal gas. These people love to move and are active, seeming restless at times. They love to talk, speak fast, and can be known to talk excessively. *Vata* types often talk with their hands. *Vatas* have a strong aversion to cold or windy conditions. Without awareness, they can have a propensity to push themselves physically beyond their limits resulting in fatigue. This *dosha* is therefore prone to tire easily and have energetic highs and lows. The *vata* immune system is the weakest of all the *doshas* and wind and cold increases their vulnerability to illness. *Vatas* are also prone to headaches.

Mentally, a *vata* is extremely creative and full of thoughts and ideas, but frequently has difficulty carrying these out. *Vata* can be "spacey", flighty, or scattered like the wind. *Vatas* tend to be indecisive, but their personalities bubble with enthusiasm and joy. *Vatas* are thinkers, introspective with thoughts always swirling around in their heads like the wind in their minds. They are adaptable to any situation, personality type, or environment. They have strong intuition, but easily become anxious or nervous. There is a tendency towards insomnia and sleep disturbance in *vata* particularly between the hours of 2-6 am. *Vatas* tend to learn very quickly, but forget things easily making them appear to be "air-heads". *Vata* is the most misunderstood of all the types, because they tend to be unconventional, having little inclination to conform. *Vata* types will tend to "beat to their own drum."

The biggest challenge *vata* types face in order to achieve their optimal weight, energy, health and vitality is their erratic appetite, and their inclination to move too much, and become exhausted. *Vata's* fast movements can make them seem awkward, clumsy or uncoordinated and make them more prone to injury. They can be picky eaters, which makes it difficult to nourish the body ideally. *Vatas* are the types who "forget" to eat, getting absorbed in a mental or physical activity so completely that they neglect the physical urges of hunger or tiredness. This inclination leads to *vata* imbalance which can make the skin, hair and nails increasingly dry, dull, and rough. *Vata* imbalance also leads to anxiety, digestive disturbances and insomnia. The frame of an imbalanced *vata* can become too thin and emaciated if there is an imbalance.

Pitta: The *pitta dosha* takes on the quality of fire. It is manifested as heat and oil in the system, the oil being the fuel feeding the flame. Characteristics that arise from *pitta's* fire qualities are sharpness, heat, light, transformation, odor, spreading and proliferation. *Pittas* are like the tiger or the rooster, which are warm-blooded, aggressive, powerful, courageous, confident, "cocky" and dominating.

Physically, a *pitta* type has an athletic, medium build with good muscle tone. They tend to have fair skin with ruddy and/or freckled complexions. Their eyes are bright, sharp, piercing and project their innate determination and focus. Their skin is more apt to develop acne, lesions and rashes. They have a confident stature about their posture. Their speech is focused, sharp, clear and concise. Their activity is purposeful and ambitious. They have a very robust appetite due to their strong digestive fire. Like the tiger, they can become fierce when they are hungry. They have strong digestion and a good metabolism. Digestively they are prone to ulcers, acidity, and indigestion. They become overheated easily, and therefore have an aversion to heat and the sun. Their immune system is strong, but they are prone to fevers, inflammation, high blood pressure and infections. They are more susceptible to inflammatory diseases than the other *doshas*.

Mentally/emotionally, *pittas* are goal-driven and competitive people. They are high achievers with great mental focus and clarity. They are passionate about what they do. They have a keen memory, and tend to be organized and efficient. *Pitta* is the only *dosha* with the power to transform. *Pitta* itself is the fire of transformation. *Pittas* take an idea and bring it into fruition with ease. They are the ones who create real and lasting change in the world. However this same fire can burn them out!

Pittas can also be controlling, ambitious, and ego driven. They often struggle with their temper and irritability. They can come across as arrogant and self-centered, and they enjoy taking "center stage" like the rooster. They are vulnerable to alcoholism, which only aggravates their fiery nature. When drinking, *pittas* may endanger themselves by showing off or engaging in quarrels. The "mean drunks" are usually *pitta* constitutions. When imbalanced, *pittas* become angry, overly aggressive, argumentative, contentious and even violent. It is an imbalanced *pitta* type who exhibits "road rage".

Being blessed with a strong metabolism and powerful digestive fire, the biggest obstacle for *pitta* types in achieving their optimal weight, health and vitality is their hearty and considerable appetite and propensity towards drinking too much alcohol which can sometimes get them into trouble. *Pittas* will build muscle easily, sometimes so easily, they can "bulk-up" undesirably with a lot of weight-bearing activity.

Kapha: The *kapha dosha* takes on the qualities of water and earth. This *dosha* is grounded, slow and deliberate, stable, dense, moist, smooth, and soft. They can be likened to the ox, cow, or elephant, exhibiting powerful strength, stamina, and steadiness. They are calm and docile, yet sometimes stubborn.

Physically, the *kapha* has a thick, sturdy frame, large strong bones and has the most strength of all the *doshas*. They have large feet and broad thick shoulders. They have well-lubricated joints, well-formed teeth, thick and lustrous hair. Their thick, oily skin wrinkles little and ages the best of all the *doshas*. *Kaphas* have large eyes with thick eye-lashes. Their hair and eyes tend to be dark brown. Mucus and phlegm tend to plague the *kapha* due to their moist watery nature. *Kaphas* have an aversion to cold, damp weather. *Kaphas* move slowly and deliberately. They tend to be more sedentary, and take more motivation to get moving, but once moving, they have the most stamina of all the *doshas*. *Kaphas* also require more sleep than *pitta* or *vata*, and are the most fertile of the *doshas* as well. They tend towards water retention, and weight accumulation. Their health vulnerabilities include pneumonia, swelling, and respiratory and congestive disorders, but they have the strongest immune system of all the *doshas*.

Mentally/emotionally the *kapha* is calm, responsible, nurturing, loyal, forgiving, and empathetic. They are generous, very family oriented, peaceful and "laid-back". They exhibit a marked sense of equilibrium. *Kaphas* make great parents and spouses and usually desire a large family. They have a greater tendency towards depression and melancholy. They also can become overly attached to people or material things. When imbalanced they become lethargic, and lazy, greedy and complacent. They can fall into "clinginess" or "hoarding", become stubborn and lack ambition.

Blessed with great skin which ages beautifully, the biggest obstacle for a *kapha* to achieve optimal weight, energy and vitality is their predisposition towards a more sedentary lifestyle, being less motivated to move and exercise. This *dosha* also requires more hours of sleep, so there are fewer hours in the day to move. *Kaphas*, like the cow, are prone to "grazing" and eating continuously all day with a constant and steady appetite. This makes a *kapha* more vulnerable to overeating. This *dosha* has a slower metabolism which is also a challenge. It will take more willpower and effort for the *kapha* to move more and eat less, but once this *dosha* is on a roll, they maintain momentum and don't give up easily. It is important to note that a *kapha* individual at their ideal weight is naturally more full-figured. Female *kaphas* tend to have full curvy hips and a fully developed chest. It is not healthy or advisable for a *kapha* to attempt to diet down into a super slim, "skinny" body type. This is not compatible with this constitution and would have a negative effect. This book is about finding your body's optimal weight and health. Thin isn't optimal or healthy for a kapha. It is important to embrace your voluptuous, curvy figure and know that is healthy for you. Self-acceptance is the new "skinny."

Although we all have some characteristics of all three *doshas, bi-doshic* people, or persons who have near equal balance of two of the *doshas,* will exhibit traits of both *doshas. Tri-doshic* persons will exhibit a balance of traits from all three *doshas.* Awareness of your tendencies and inclinations is a step towards enlightenment. By recognizing your own pitfalls and predispositions you are better able to make a firm commitment to doing what helps you look and feel your best and stay in balance.

Focus for Today: Let the awareness of your *dosha* type fuel your compassion for yourself and your predispositions. Also let this awareness focus and direct you towards changes that benefit your *dosha* type, leading you towards maximum health, energy, youthfulness, weight and vitality.

Journal: What have you learned about yourself that will better enable you to make the best choices for your health, weight, energy and vitality? Are you surprised by the results of your *dosha* quiz? How will knowing your type change the way you take care of yourself mentally and physically? Do you recognize the other types in those around you? How will knowing their type affect your interactions with these people? How will knowing your type and their types make you more compassionate to others and to yourself?

Recipe of the Day:

Chai-Cashew Smoothie

(Makes 1 serving)

1 organic chai tea bag
6 oz water
1 Tbsp cashew butter
Agave nectar to taste

Heat the water and steep the tea bag. Place the cashew butter in a blender and add the concentrated chai tea. Add agave to taste, and blend for a nice warm smoothie perfect for the winter months! In summer, feel free to add a bit of ice and blend.

Daily Food Journal

Date:_____ Intention for the day:_____ Weight:_____

Water: ☐☐☐⬛⬛⬛⬛⬛ *X off one water for every 8 oz. of water that you drink. This includes lemon waters. During a cleanse you should have at least 3 lemon waters daily.*

YOGI PLATE	➡	¼ Protein ➡ ⬅ ½ Veggies ¼ Whole Grains ➡

Rate your hunger, mood, energy

and after meal satisfaction

1=Low   2=Average   3=High

Time	Meal/ Snack	Food/ Beverage	Hungry?	Mood?	Energy?	Satisfied?
	Breakfast					
	Snack					
	Lunch					
	Snack					
	Dinner					
	Snack					

At the end of the day, reflect on how many servings you had of the following foods/beverages:

Vegetables (Unlimited)	
Whole Grains (Women 1 -3)	
Fruit (Aim for 2)	
Protein (Aim for 3 or more)	

Did I Avoid?	Yes	No	How Much?
Alcohol			
Soft Drinks			
White Sugar			
Artificial Sweeteners			
Processed Food			
Fast Food			

Alert! Use Meat Sparingly

Consume meat no more than 3 times a week!

List your observations and insights for the day. These include successes and behaviors that need attention:

_____
_____
_____
_____
_____

Day 15: Diet by *Dosha*

We now know that we are not created exactly the same. Each of us is born with a specific *dosha* type or set of constitutional characteristics that define our personality as well as our physical body. It is not a stretch then to conclude that individual dietary needs may vary according to our constitution. More specialized eating for our type best serves our health, weight, energy and vitality. Although most quality foods are healthful for all the *doshas*, there are some specific eating recommendations by *dosha* to optimize health and balance. Eating according to your *dosha* can be quite complex, but I have attempted to simplify this and make it as easy as possible. If you would like a more in-depth breakdown of eating by the *dosha*, I recommend <u>Ayurveda: A Life of Balance</u> by Maya Tiwari.

Vata: *Vata dosha* is nurtured by eating foods that are warm, moist, oily, sweet, salty and sour. Root vegetables and soups are particularly nourishing and balancing to *vata*. *Vata*, which is the easiest *dosha* to become disturbed or unbalanced, can be aggravated by foods which are cold, dry or gassy. Because of *vata*'s cold, dry and restless tendencies, dried fruit, crackers, chips, dry toast, white sugar, and too many raw foods are not recommended. A completely raw-foods diet is not for *vata*, as this diet can send it quickly out of balance, leading to hyperactivity, insomnia, scattered thinking, anxiety and nervousness. Seventy percent of the foods in the diet of a *vata* should be cooked, except during the summer when it is warm and humid, and then *vata* can eat more raw foods. Fifty percent raw can be OK for *vata* during hot, humid weather, but this can vary according to the individual. As a *vata*, I can attest to this myself. Personally, when I eat too much raw produce, I tend to notice disturbed sleep and overall agitation.

During spring, fall, and winter, soups are very soothing and warming to *vata* and help replace some much needed moisture. Stir-frys are balancing to *vata* as well. Fresh juicy fruits replenish *vata*'s dry system, and are very nourishing. Nuts and seeds of all kinds help balance *vata*. They have both a warming quality about them, and are a great source of oil, which is very beneficial to *vata*'s dry system. In general, the use of oils, including *ghee* in a *vata* diet is very helpful. Legumes can be difficult for *vata*'s delicate digestive system, exacerbating *vata*'s gassy nature, thus large quantities of beans should be avoided. Non-GMO tofu and lentils are fine in moderation. Carbonated beverages also aggravate *vata*'s already gassy nature. Salt is balancing for *vata*, and helps hold moisture in the body. All forms of dairy products are nourishing to *vata*'s mind-body system. Warming spices such as cinnamon, cardamom, ginger, and black pepper are very harmonizing for *vata*. Hot peppers, although warming, can be difficult for the vulnerable digestive system of a *vata*, and can cause agitation, restlessness and scattered thinking.

Pitta: Of all the *doshas, pitta* is the most nourished by sweet tasting foods. Use any natural sweeteners other than white sugar. Most fresh fruits, whole grains and whole grain breads are strengthening and harmonizing to *pitta* as well. *Pitta* does very well with raw foods since they have the strongest digestive fire of all the *doshas*. Raw foods practically cook themselves in the intense digestive fire once ingested by a *pitta*. *Pitta* digests almost all legumes well (except lentils), and they are a great source of fiber and protein as well as carbohydrates for this *dosha*. Eating plenty of grains and legumes is a great way to satiate *pitta*'s tremendous appetite. *Ghee* and butter are ideal. Other oils should be used in moderation in light of the fact that this *dosha* is very oily by nature. Seeds and nuts should be used in moderation because of their high oil content and their heating qualities. These also tend to be highly salted which further inflames *pitta*. The best option for *pitta* is to use unsalted raw nuts and seeds as opposed to roasted or cooked, which are more heating to their system. Warming spices and hot peppers also aggravate *pitta*, bringing out temper and more aggressive tendencies and increase internal heat, which is irritating to *pitta*. Cool foods and drinks are best for *pitta*. Soups can be overly warming. *Pitta* does well with milk, butter, cheese and *ghee*, but sour dairy products intensify the already acidic digestive system of a *pitta*. They should avoid sour cream, buttermilk, cottage cheese, and sour yogurt. Use cheese in moderation, due to its oily, salty and often sour nature. Sour fruits, including tomatoes, also create excess acidity for *pitta*. Eat sweeter fruits, and wait until fruits are at the peak of ripeness to ingest. Overly acidic foods like vinegar, pickles, sour kraut are aggravating to *pitta*. Meat, particularly red meat, promotes anger and aggression in a *pitta type*. It is best to minimize or eliminate red meat and eat white meats only in moderation. Deep fried foods intensify *pitta*, as can seafood. These should also be eaten in moderation. As discussed earlier, alcoholic beverages tend to increase and exaggerate *pitta* tendencies.

Kapha: Due to the excess phlegm and mucous that characterizes the *kapha* constitution; dairy products are not helpful to this *dosha*. Dairy promotes phlegm, and will exacerbate congestion and water retention for *kapha*. Low—fat milk in moderation (preferably boiled first) and *ghee* are the only cow dairy products recommended for *kapha*. Goat's milk and goat cheese are suggested as the optimal substitute for cow's milk and cheese. Light meals loaded with an assortment of vegetables suit *kapha* well, preventing this *dosha* from feeling weighted down, however *kapha* needs warm, dry food to counteract the damp, cold nature that plagues this *dosha*, particularly in winter and spring. *Kapha* especially benefits from light fruits such as apples or pears. *Kapha* does well with fewer sweeteners, due to their propensity to gain weight easily. Honey is the sweetener of choice for *kapha*, particularly raw honey which is said to balance *kapha*. *Kapha* does well with all legumes and dried fruits. Hot spices such as cayenne help to stimulate *kapha*s and get them moving, so these are recommended. Nuts and seeds need to be eaten very sparingly due to their density and heaviness which bring out this aspect of *kapha*'s nature too. Also, nuts and seeds can promote weight gain in *kapha*. *Kapha*s need to go easy on all oils due to their heaviness, and tendency to weigh down the system. Oil may also promote weight accumulation for *kapha*. Salt should be used sparingly as well. *Kapha* has a strong predisposition towards water retention, and salt can exacerbate this, making *kapha*s look heavier than they actually are. This *dosha* can eat a combination of cooked and raw foods, with a stronger emphasis on raw foods during the warm summer months. Keep meals light and include things like salads, and fresh fruits. *Kapha*s want to avoid foods like red meat and hot cereals which make them feel heavy, weighted down and dull their energy. In general *kapha* types need to reduce overall food intake. They should eat smaller meals and avoid "grazing" between meals. This *dosha* is most prone to weight gain and overall tissue increase.

Each season of the year takes on the qualities of one of the *doshas*. In the west, spring tends to be cool and damp and is considered *kapha* season. Summer is hot and and takes on *pitta's* fire nature. Fall and winter are cold, dry and windy which are considered *vata* in quality. These seasons have a powerful affect on the balance of our own *doshas*. Most people are affected by the qualities of the seasons, and need to adjust their eating accordingly. Bi-doshic individuals do well to modify their diet by season.

Vata-Pitta: Fall and winter, are considered *vata* season because of their cold, dry, windy qualities. During this time, *vata* is more easily thrown out of balance for a *vata-pitta* constitution. Therefore it is best to follow a *vata*-balancing diet during this time of year. During spring and summer it is recommended to follow a *pitta*-balancing diet. Due to the warm, heating qualities of these seasons, it is more likely that *pitta* qualities will become more dominant.

Vata-Kapha: A *vata* balancing diet should be followed in summer and fall because the cold, dry, windy aspect of this season can aggravate *vata*. Late winter and early spring is *kapha* season. Due to the cool, damp, heavy nature of this time of year, the *kapha* aspect of your nature is more easily imbalanced. A *kapha* balancing diet is recommended for this part of the year.

Pitta-Kapha: Follow the *pitta*-pacifying diet during late spring, summer, and fall. During these seasons, your *pitta* is more easily deranged or imbalanced due to the warming qualities of these seasons. During winter and early spring, *kapha* is more likely to become imbalanced due to the cool, heavy, damp nature of the season. It is therefore recommended that you follow a *kapha* balancing diet during this time.

Vata-Pitta-Kapha (tri-doshic): During fall through mid-winter, *vata* season, it is best to follow the *vata*-balancing dietary recommendations. From late winter through early spring, follow a *kapha*-balancing diet, and from late spring through summer, eating a *pitta*-pacifying diet best serves you.

As a strong *vata dosha* with *pitta* being a distant second, I find that I am able to navigate somewhat towards a *pitta* diet during the *pitta* season of summer. It is this time of year when I find myself eating many more raw foods. However, if I eat more than 50% raw, I notice signs of *vata* imbalance emerge such as waking up in the night, restless sleeping, more nervous fidgety energy, worry or anxiety and difficulty sitting in meditation. In the summer months, I suggest all *doshas* eat at least one raw meal a day so that you receive the benefits all the nutrients and enzymes contained in raw fruits, vegetables, seeds and nuts, while helping to keep *pitta* in balance. Fortunately, during this time of year there is an abundance of delicious raw produce grown locally. We discovered in our *dosha* quiz that we all contain some proportion of all of the *doshas*. We all can and should adapt the *doshas* toward the season we are in, as we cannot underestimate the influence the seasonal *dosha* can have upon our own inner balance.

Below you will find a list of foods which either support or imbalance each *dosha*. Ayurvedic diet for the *dosha* can become extremely complex, but I have tried to simplify it to make it as user friendly as possible.

Vata Balancing Foods	*Vata* Disturbing Foods
All organic dairy	Caffeinated drinks
All natural sweeteners in moderation	Red meat
Fresh, juicy fruits	White sugar
Root vegetables	Bitter greens
Warming spices	Raw vegetables (moderation only)
Cooked vegetables	Legumes
Nuts	Iced beverages
Seeds	Cold foods
Mung or soy beans	Dried fruits
Warm cereals	Carbonated beverages
Tofu/organic soy (in moderation)	Crackers, granola, corn chips, dry foods
Soups	Cruciferous vegetables such as cabbage, brocoli, Brussels sprouts, etc.
Stir frys	Mushrooms
Heated foods	
White meat in moderation	

Seafood in moderation	
Wheat, oats, rice	
Eggs	

Pitta Balancing Foods   *Pitta* Disturbing Foods

Pitta Balancing Foods	*Pitta* Disturbing Foods
Milk, butter, ghee	Hot or spicy foods
Natural sweeteners (molasses and honey are less favorable, raw honey OK)	Vinegar, pickled foods or sour foods
Raw fruits and vegetables	Seafood, shellfish
All legumes	Lentils
Most oils in moderation, butter and ghee are ideal	Red meat
Cool foods and drinks	Deep fried foods
Whole grain breads	Sour fruits
Most whole grains	Sour dairy: sour cream, buttermilk, cottage cheese, sour yogurt
Fresh water fish	Alcoholic beverages
White meat in moderation	White sugar
Eggs	Garlic, onions
Coconut, raw nuts, sunflower seeds	Roasted, salted nuts, salty, deep-fried chips

Kapha Balancing Foods   *Kapha* Disturbing Foods

Kapha Balancing Foods	*Kapha* Disturbing Foods
Most legumes, soy, tofu	Black lentils
Boiled, low-fat organic milk	Avocado
Goat's milk and cheese, soy milk and cheese, and butter products, buttermilk, ghee	Cow's milk/dairy
Raw fruits, apples, pears, berries	Hot cereals
Raw vegetables	Red meat
Raw honey or stevia	Fish
Heating spices	Tofu
Legumes	Heavy oils

Bitter greens	Kidney beans
Whole grains	Salt
Sunflower seeds and pumpkin seeds	Nuts, use sparingly
White meat in moderation	Overcooked foods
Eggs	Rice, basmati ok in moderation
Light oils in moderation such as corn oil, canola oil, sunflower oil or safflower oil	Heavy oils: peanut oil, olive oil, sesame oil, coconut oil, avocado oil
Dried fruits, dry foods like whole-grain toast, granola, whole grain crackers	bananas, sweet melons

Focus for Today: Begin to tweak your eating to better support your *dosha*.

Journal: When you read about diet for your particular constitutional type, were there any surprises? Were there foods you have already noticed do and don't agree with you?

Recipe of the Day: This recipe is suitable for all of the *doshas*.

Veggie Quiche

(6 servings)

Crust:

1 cup whole wheat pastry flour
¼ cup ground flax seeds
½ stick butter or ¼ cup *ghee*
½ tsp sea salt
5 Tbsp. water

Mix and press into pie pan. Use fork to puncture bottom of crust in several places, and prebake the crust 10 min. at 400.

Veggies:

3 cloves garlic, minced
½ large onion, chopped
½ zucchini, chopped
½ red bell pepper, chopped
½ yellow squash, chopped

Sauté the veggies until soft, in 1 tablespoon of olive oil.

Custard:

3 organic eggs
1 cup organic half and half
Salt and pepper

Whisk ingredients together.

¾ cup cheese of your choice optional

Place cheese in prebaked pie crust. Place sautéed veggies on top of the cheese. Pour egg mixture over the veggies. Bake 45 min at 375.

Daily Food Journal

Date:_____ Intention for the day:_____ Weight:_____

Water: *X off one water for every 8 oz. of water that you drink. This includes lemon waters. During a cleanse you should have at least 3 lemon waters daily.*

| YOGI PLATE | ➡ | ¼ Protein ➡ | ⊕ | ⬅ ½ Veggies |
| | | ¼ Whole Grains ➡ | | |

Rate your hunger, mood, energy and after meal satisfaction

1=Low   2=Average   3=High

Time	Meal/ Snack	Food/ Beverage	Hungry?	Mood?	Energy?	Satisfied?
	Breakfast					
	Snack					
	Lunch					
	Snack					
	Dinner					
	Snack					

At the end of the day, reflect on how many servings you had of the following foods/beverages:

Vegetables (Unlimited)	
Whole Grains (Women 1 -3)	
Fruit (Aim for 2)	
Protein (Aim for 3 or more)	

Did I Avoid?	Yes	No	How Much?
Alcohol			
Soft Drinks			
White Sugar			
Artificial Sweeteners			
Processed Food			
Fast Food			

Alert! Use Meat Sparingly

Consume meat no more than 3 times a week!

List your observations and insights for the day. These include successes and behaviors that need attention:

_____
_____
_____
_____
_____

Day 16: Yoga by *Dosha*

Ayurvedic philosophy holds Yoga in highest regard as a system for maintaining health and well-being and for treating specific ailments. Yoga is considered the ideal system of exercises for maintaining optimal health. In Ayurveda, any imbalance of the mind, body or spirit can be attributed to the accumulation or excess of one of the three *doshas* in the body. It is when one of the *doshas* becomes disturbed and imbalanced that we are vulnerable to disease. Regular Yoga practice can have a powerful balancing effect on all of the *doshas*. However, there are times when a specific Yoga practice is needed in order to bring a specific *dosha* into balance. Most often, it is a person's dominant *dosha* which is most likely to become disturbed. However, it is possible for any *dosha* to accumulate in the system causing an imbalance in that particular *dosha* even if it is not a person's dominant *dosha*.

The seasons have a powerful effect on the *doshas*. Fall and winter are considered *vata* in nature because of the cold, dry and windy conditions which correspond with the air and ether qualities of *vata*. These qualities in nature also increase our own *vata* qualities. Late winter and early spring are considered *kapha* in nature because of the dampness of the melting snow and the spring rains and the cooler temperatures, which correspond with the earth and water qualities of *kapha*. During this time of year our own *kapha* tendencies are increased. Summer is considered *pitta* season, due to the heating, fire-like qualities inherent in summer. During the summer months, our own *pitta* qualities are exacerbated. What are the specific Yoga practice needs for the *doshas*? How do you know if one of the *doshas* has come out of balance? How can Yoga bring each *dosha* back into balance?

Vata

Vata types benefit greatly from a regular Yoga practice. It calms their anxious nervous tendencies, helps them enjoy better quality sleep and teaches them to move with more balance and coordination. *Vata's* light bird-like bones make inversions readily accessible in Yoga practice. Caution though, as *vata* tends to lack coordination. *Vatas* on the whole have the least flexibility of all the *doshas*. The dry quality of their nature tends to dry out the joints making them more prone to stiff joints and arthritis. *Vata* types also tend to move too much and too quickly, which can be detrimental to their Yoga practice, making them vulnerable to injury. A well-designed Yoga practice can help *vata* types learn to slow down. It is best for *vata* types to move slowly and gracefully, and take time to warm and lubricate the joints as they come to their Yoga practice. Longer held poses well-serve this *dosha*. *Vata's* erratic energy levels can be challenging when incorporating a Yoga practice into their routine. It is important for them to honor their present energy level and tailor their Yoga practice to their body's needs. Restorative Yoga is a great alternative for times when energy is low. Moist heat is also helpful when *vata* types practice Yoga.

Do You Have a *Vata* Imbalance?

Vata, which translates literally as "wind", is the force that governs fall and winter months according to Yoga and Ayurveda. It is *vata* that brings on the dryness, cold, wind and stiffness during the winter months. Because of the extreme nature of winter in many parts of the country, many people will find that their own internal *vata* qualities have been thrown off balance during this time of year. Too many raw foods, anxiety, lack of sleep, travel, and exposure to windy conditions can also increase *vata* in the system leading to a *vata* disturbance. When a *vata* imbalance is not corrected, over time one can begin to experience chills, tremors, icy cold extremities, emaciation, constipation, insomnia, rough, dry skin, anxiety, clumsiness, mental confusion, and arthritis.

Take this self-assessment quiz to see if you are experiencing a *vata* imbalance. (*Note: These questions came to me via Kristin Bjarnason, RN, RYT 500.)

1. Is your skin dryer than usual, itching or taut?
2. Are your lips chapped?
3. Do your throat and nasal passages feel dry?
4. Is your hair dry and does it have more spilt-ends?
5. Have you felt more forgetful, foggy, or spaced out?
6. Has your digestion been irregular?
7. Do you notice more abdominal gas or constipation?
8. Have you noticed stiffness in the muscles and joints?
9. Have you had increased cracking and popping in your joints?
10. Have you had difficulty focusing?
11. Have you felt more fretful, anxious, or worried than usual?
12. Have you had difficulty sleeping or more restless sleep?
13. Is your mind full of chatter, jumping from one thought to the next?
14. Do you have a dry cough?

If you answered "yes" to several of these questions, it is a sign that your own *vata* qualities may have accumulated in your body creating a *vata* imbalance.

Vata Balancing Yoga Practice:

Vata is the *dosha* which can most easily become deranged or out of balance. *Vata dosha* governs the other *doshas*, so when it becomes deranged, the other *doshas* can more easily come out of balance as well. To re-balance disturbed *vata*, balancing poses work well to recreate a sense of balance in the mind and cultivate inner stillness. In a *vata* balancing practice, it is important to warm the body with warming *pranayamas* or Yogic breathing techniques and Yoga poses, and to practice in a warm room or environment.

Vata is considered a *vayu* or wind which can often blow erratically. Moving more slowly and steadily from posture to posture keeps from further aggravating *vata*. A *vata* balancing Yoga practice should avoid quick movements and transitions, fast pulsating or loud music, and jumping forward and back in sun salutations. Sun salutations, if practiced, should move slowly and rhythmically.

In a *vata* balancing Yoga practice it is important to incorporate a joint-lubricating warm–up, because *vata* accumulates in the joints causing stiffness and cracking of the joints. Because *vata* qualities are that of air and ether, a *vata* imbalance brings about a sense of ungroundedness and instability. Focus on grounding poses such as triangle, Hindi squat, mountain pose, tree pose, and child's pose. Any pose which keeps you on the ground or close to the ground calms *vata*. Forward folds and gentle twists of any kind calm the central nervous system. *Vata* imbalance is known to create nervousness and anxiety. To create a deeper sense of stability it will help to use an earth-bound *drishti* or focal point, and in standing poses root the big toes and pinky toes firmly into the floor. A balancing breath such as *nadi shodhana* or a warming breath such as *ujjai*, are particularly useful *pranayama*s or yogic breathing techniques for rebalancing *vata*.

Kapha

*Kapha*s need a more challenging, "sweaty" exercise regime and Yoga practice to balance their slower metabolism and more sedentary predisposition. *Kapha*s tend to be the most flexible of all the *doshas*, and they have the benefit of supple, well-lubricated joints. *Kapha*s have the strongest, steadiest physical endurance of all three *doshas*. Their downfall is their lack of motivation, tendency towards complacency and lethargy, and their sporadic, "hit or miss pattern" of exercise and Yoga practice. This can make them susceptible to injury and weight gain. However, once motivated, *kapha* surpasses the other *doshas* in strength, flexibility and endurance.

Do You Have a *Kapha* Imbalance?

Kapha takes on the qualities of water and earth. It is moist, cool, heavy and solid. When water and earth come together mud is formed. It is the qualities of *kapha* which give the body form and cohesion. Too much *kapha* can weigh the body down causing it to be sluggish and lethargic. *Kapha* can clog the system with mucus and water retention. Late winter and early spring is the season in which we are most prone to the influence of *kapha* qualities. Left unresolved, a *kapha* imbalance can lead to depression, weight gain, lethargy, sluggishness, fatigue, pale skin, heavy congestion, water retention, and over-sleeping. Take the following quiz to determine whether you have a *kapha* imbalance:

1. Have you felt sluggish and lethargic?
2. Have you had a runny nose or felt congested?
3. Have you experienced weight gain?
4. Do you feel an aversion to cool damp air?
5. Have you noticed water retention?
6. Have you experienced a feeling of melancholy over the last few weeks?
7. Have you been more emotional lately? Cry easily?
8. Have you noticed you are nibbling or grazing more often?
9. Have you been sleepier than normal?
10. Do you feel a bit stagnated?
11. Do you feel you have been lacking in motivation in recent weeks?
12. Are you experiencing a phlegmy cough?
13. Do you feel as if you are moving slower than normal?

If you have answered "yes" to several of these questions, then you are experiencing the symptoms of increased *kapha* qualities.

Kapha Balancing Yoga Practice:

Yoga practice is a great way to rebalance the heaviness of *kapha* and get things moving. A *kapha* balancing Yoga practice begins with mind clearing, warming *pranayama*, or Yoga breathing. *Kapalabhati* is a great breathing technique for clearing the sinuses, and is said to clear the mind and help reduce excess weight gained over the winter months. It is not appropriate for people with high blood pressure, pregnancy, glaucoma or heart disease. *Surya bhedana* is a great alternative for people with these challenges. *Surya bhedana* is a warming energizing Yoga breath which involves breathing in through the right nostril and out through the left.

The *kapha* balancing *asana* practice is enhanced by energizing, motivating music. When practicing for *kapha* rebalance, the *drishti* should be above the horizon. The practice should be playful, full of joy and laughter. It starts low to the ground due to the heavy nature and groundedness of *kapha*. The practice slowly builds in intensity, with the intent to invigorate the mind and body and to rev up the metabolism. Longer held poses help increase stamina, and create a detoxifying sweat. Poses such as backbends to open the chest are encouraged since they invigorate, as well as cultivate joy and openness. Forward bending is minimized since it tends to calm and slow the nervous system. Headstand if appropriate is excellent to balance *kapha*. Headstand is not recommended for people with high blood pressure, glaucoma, or pregnancy.

Practice with these things in mind, and find yourself feeling your *kapha* qualities are more balanced!

Pitta

Pitta types are strong and athletic, focused and goal oriented. They have moderate flexibility. They tend to be very consistent in their Yoga practice and exercise regime. However, this *dosha* can bring too much competition, force, and over-muscling into Yoga. They often mistakenly turn Yoga practice into a competition, comparing themselves with others and going to extremes to out-do them. In general, *pitta doshas* tend to be overly intense about any activity or project they take on and this comes into play when they practice Yoga. *Pittas* may try to force themselves into a pose they are not ready for. Being overly ambitious and ego driven along with a tendency to over-muscle a Yoga pose makes *pitta* prone to injury in Yoga practice. Although pitas are attracted to the more athletic and power forms of Yoga, they actually benefit more from a calming and cooling style of Yoga. "Hot Yoga" and "power Yoga" are not for the already fiery *pitta*, and these styles of Yoga will only aggravate and imbalance this *dosha*.

Do You Have a *Pitta* Imbalance?

Pitta qualities correspond with the element of fire and consist of heat, oil, spreading, odor, light, sharpness, and proliferation. People of a *pitta* constitution are more likely to suffer from an inbalance of this *dosha*, but under the right circumstances any constitution can experience a *pitta* imbalance. Some things which can lead to accumulation of *pitta* might be exposure to extreme heat, a diet of salty, oily, spicy foods, a demanding career, or a diet high in acidity.

According to Ayurveda, summer is *pitta* season. When exposed to extreme heat for a duration of time, our own fire-like qualities can become exacerbated and out of balance. If *pitta* imbalance is not corrected, one may experience increased hunger and thirst, rashes and inflammation, irritability, anger, excessive indigestion, ulcers, yellow skin and eyes and ultimately inflammatory diseases. Take the following quiz to determine whether or not your own inherent *pitta* or fire qualities have been aggravated:

1. Have you felt overheated?
2. Have you noticed indigestion or stomach acidity?
3. Have your skin and hair become oilier?
4. Have you been experiencing rashes or acne?
5. Have you observed an increased appetite?
6. Have you observed a slight weight gain?
7. Have you suffered from allergies or inflammation of any kind?
8. Do you feel more aggressive or have more "drive" than usual?
9. Have you noticed your temper flare more than usual?
10. Do you feel irritated by things that wouldn't ordinarily bother you?
11. Have you notice increased sweating accompanied by a stronger odor than usual?
12. Do you feel an aversion to heat or direct sun?
13. Have you experienced increased thirst?
14. Have your bowel movements been more loose than usual?

If you find yourself answering "yes" to several of these questions, then your own *pitta* or fire element has come out of balance.

Pitta Balancing Yoga Practice:

Yoga practice is a great way to re-balance the *pitta dosha*. Begin your Yoga practice with cooling *pranayama* (Yoga breaths) such as *chandra bhedana*, *sitali* or *sitkari*. These breathing techniques should be learned from a professional Yoga instructor.

Practice moon salutations as opposed to super-heating sun salutations.

Although a *pitta* balancing practice should be a more cooling "lunar" practice, it is also important to "quench" the inner fire a bit without over-heating it. Therefore one can incorporate some more heating poses into the practice without going overboard and over-muscling the poses. Relaxing melodious music is helpful in creating the optimal setting. I suggest half-moon, crescent moon, and triangle. Forward bending also calms and cools *pitta*. A *pitta* balancing practice should include plenty of forward folds, both standing and seated. Plow and shoulder-stand are perfect *pitta* calming inversions. Gentle twists should be included to calm and cool the central nervous system. Restorative crescent moon on a bolster finishes the practice with a cooling lunar nature before ending the practice in *viparita karani* (supported legs up the wall using blankets under the sit-bones.)

The key to a *pitta* balancing Yoga practice is that it is cooling, calming, relaxing, yet has enough vigor to quench the fire already there. Give the fire something to feed on without igniting it further. Practicing in this manner daily should cool the inner fire that has been aggravated by the summer heat!

Yoga and Ayurveda work in conjunction to keep the *doshas* in balance and harmony. Once you recognize a *dosha* imbalance, it is important to turn to the naturally harmonizing sister sciences of Yoga and Ayurveda.

Focus for Today: Find time to do a Yoga practice that balances your *dosha*.

Journal: When practicing Yoga for your specific *dosha* imbalance, what did you notice? How did you feel during and after practice?

Recipe of the Day:

Quinoa Salad with Walnuts and Roasted Grapes

(Serves large group)

2 cups organic quinoa
4 cups water
¼ cup extra virgin olive oil
1 small red onion, chopped
2 cups organic red grapes
1 cup chopped walnuts
1 cup crumbled Feta
Large handful chopped Italian parsley

The Dressing:

Juice of 1 lemon or ¼ cup red wine vinegar
3 to 4 cloves garlic
Hand-full of fresh basil leaves
¼ cup extra virgin olive oil
Sea salt and pepper to taste
½ cup organic red grapes (to add sweetness)

Cook the quinoa in the water until water is evaporated. Let cool to room temperature. Coat grapes in the extra virgin olive oil and roast in oven at 425 for 10 to 12 minutes. Mix red onion, roasted grapes, walnuts, parsley and feta into cooled quinoa. Mix together the dressing ingredients into a blender and liquefy. Pour over quinoa and gently mix into salad. Chill in refrigerator.

Daily Food Journal

Date:_____   Intention for the day:_____   Weight:_____

Water: [cup][cup][cup][cup][cup][cup][cup][cup]   *X off one water for every 8 oz. of water that you drink. This includes lemon waters. During a cleanse you should have at least 3 lemon waters daily.*

YOGI PLATE →   ¼ Protein   ½ Veggies   ¼ Whole Grains

	Rate your hunger, mood, energy and after meal satisfaction		
1=Low	2=Average		3=High

Time	Meal/ Snack	Food/ Beverage	Hungry?	Mood?	Energy?	Satisfied?
	Breakfast					
	Snack					
	Lunch					
	Snack					
	Dinner					
	Snack					

At the end of the day, reflect on how many servings you had of the following foods/beverages:

Vegetables (Unlimited)	
Whole Grains (Women 1 -3)	
Fruit (Aim for 2)	
Protein (Aim for 3 or more)	

Did I Avoid?	Yes	No	How Much?
Alcohol			
Soft Drinks			
White Sugar			
Artificial Sweeteners			
Processed Food			
Fast Food			

Alert! Use Meat Sparingly
Consume meat no more than 3 times a week!

List your observations and insights for the day. These include successes and behaviors that need attention:

_____
_____
_____
_____
_____

Day 17: The Six Tastes

In Ayurveda, taste is believed to have as much effect on the mind-body system as the food itself. Ayurveda recognizes six tastes, and each taste in itself brings out various characteristics—physically, mentally, emotionally and spiritually. The six tastes are: sweet, salty, sour, bitter, pungent and astringent.

Sweet taste: This taste is considered the most nourishing and *sattvic* taste in Ayurveda. This is because some of the most nourishing foods from nature are sweet, such as fresh fruits and vegetables, and milk (which is the first form of nourishment we receive in life). Sweet taste is the taste of sustenance. Sweet taste is said to nourish and build the body's tissues. Too much sweet taste increases or enlarges the body tissues beyond their ideal size, and promotes phlegm, congestion and even lethargy. Sweet taste corresponds with and increases "sweet" emotions such as joy and love, and it promotes a feeling of contentment. Stress tends to send us craving sweet taste, because we are seeking the overall sense of "sweetness" this taste imparts. Sweet taste also increases energy. Often people crave this taste during energy lows. This taste is nourishing to all three *doshas*, but *kapha* needs less sweet taste due to its predisposition to build bodily tissue. Sweet taste increases *kapha* and is considered a tissue developer in Ayurveda. Sweet taste should be enjoyed in moderation, if one is not looking to increase in size. *Vata* benefits enormously from sweet taste because it is very grounding to *vata*'s wind-like, restless, nervous tendencies. Sweet taste balances *pitta* well because of its cooling nature, quieting *pitta*'s "fire" a bit. People suffering from depression tend to crave sweet taste in order to bring their emotional state back into balance, because it brings out pleasant feelings such as love and "nourishment". However, this craving can be at the root of the typical weight gain known to accompany depression. If you find that you are incorporating large amounts of sweet taste into your diet and wish to lose weight, it is a good idea to gradually reduce it in quantity. Slowly decreasing sweeteners and sweet foods will increase the tongue's sensitivity to sweet taste in smaller amounts. Some sweet taste is important and necessary for harmony and wellbeing, but in excess, it causes build up of tissue and *ama*.

Salty taste: When this taste is achieved through sources other than table salt, salty taste usually contains beneficial minerals. It is *rajasic* in nature, as it stimulates the senses. It is helpful to all the *doshas* in small amounts, but is most beneficial to *vata*. This is because salty taste is warming and increases water retention, and *vata* is most apt to be cold and dry. Salty taste is good for the joints, as it keeps them moist and lubricated, and it helps keep the body's electrolytes in balance. Too much salty taste can be aggravating to *pitta*, creating too much heat. *Kapha* needs salty taste the least because of its tendency to retain fluids. Too much salty taste for a *kapha* can lead to hypertension, water weight gain, and swelling. This taste is also considered a tissue builder in Ayurveda. On the emotional level, salty taste creates zest for life, and encourages confidence and courage. Salt itself is a mild sedative. However, in excessive amounts, salty taste fosters greed and attachment. It is important to note that salty taste is powerful in very small amounts. Small amounts stimulate digestion, but large amounts can stimulate vomiting. Because processed "table salt" is extremely concentrated in taste and lacks the accompanying minerals, it is best to receive this taste from mineral salts or sea salts.

Sour taste: This taste is appropriate for all of the *doshas* in small amounts. It is rajasic, or stimulating in nature. This taste aids in digestion, and helps rid the body of accumulated toxins, and relieves constipation. Sour taste has a warming quality. *Vata* benefits most from sour taste because of its warming quality and because of its benefits to the digestive system, which in *vata* tends to be a bit inconsistent. It is important to know that this taste is said to increase the appetite. *Pitta* can be adversely affected by sour taste because it can increase the already strong appetite characteristic of *pitta*. Sour taste can aggravate *pitta* because of its heating, "burning" nature, and it can increase indigestion and heartburn. Also, *pitta* has a stronger tendancy towards stomach acidity and ulcers. Citrus fruits, yogurt, buttermilk, sour cream, cottage cheese, vinegar, and unripe fruits tend to increase *pitta*, therefore these should be eaten in moderation, and fruits should be eaten in the peak of ripeness by the *pitta dosha* to reduce sour taste. *Kapha* is increased by sour taste, and it will exaggerate *kapha*'s already steady appetite, so *kapha* should use sour taste in moderation as well. In excess, this taste can produce body aches and cramps. Emotionally, excess sour taste is said to promote a "sour" disposition. However, sour taste is a mild stimulant and can help relieve depression.

Bitter taste: In Ayurveda, this taste is known to be detoxifying to the body. It cleanses the liver, blood and aids in digestion. Bitter taste reduces body fat, but in excess, can deplete the tissues, causing emaciation and severe dryness. Bitter taste can calm the stomach and ease digestive discomfort. This taste is considered *tamasic* because of its reducing, depleting nature. However, this taste is necessary in differing amounts for each of the *doshas*. It is the least helpful to *vata* due to its cooling effects and its tendency to reduce the bodily tissues, and *vata* leans towards coldness and a lean frame. Bitter taste is helpful to *pitta* because the inherent coolness in bitter taste helps balance excess heat and it aids in calming "firey" digestion. Indigestion and hyperacidity is often a problem for *pitta*. *Kapha* is benefitted by bitter taste because it helps with weight reduction, and helps alleviate dullness and lethargy. Mentally and emotionally, in the right doses, bitter taste is said to open the mind and increase consciousness. In excess, it can foster feelings of disconnection, hyperactivity or nervousness, which will quickly aggravate *vata*. Considerable amounts of bitter taste can increase feelings of grief, loneliness and bitterness itself. Bitter tasting foods include leafy greens, coffee, cocoa and turmeric.

Pungent taste: This taste is stimulating. It is found in foods like garlic, hot peppers, ginger, cinnamon, onion, radishes and mustard. Pungent taste is considered *rajasic* due to its stimulating nature. This taste is warming, increases circulation, and promotes sweating. It is purported to help liquefy body fat, and to expel it from the body as well as to increase the metabolism, but it also increases appetite. Pungent taste is least beneficial for *pitta* because of its heating, sweat inducing and appetite stimulating properties. Although pungent taste is warming, which is of benefit to *vata*, its drying and stimulating effects are not as advantageous to this *dosha*. *Kapha* benefits from the stimulating effects of pungent taste as well as its fat reducing properties and its drying effect. It is particularly effective on drying out the sinuses.

Mentally and emotionally, pungent taste is said to promote clarity, move stagnation, and increase motivation. It is used medicinally to help alleviate depression because it is said to arouse the mind and the senses, rev-up the nervous system and kindle enthusiasm. It is also used to help "burn away" toxins and congestion. In excess this taste can encourage restlessness, agitation, insomnia, and anxiety. Too much of this taste can also create inflammation, heartburn, diarrhea, and ulcers. Emotionally, overindulgence in this taste can nurture hatred and anger.

Astringent taste: This taste is primarily used medicinally. It has contractive qualities, which can constrict blood vessels and help stop bleeding and promote clotting. It can also stop diarrhea and excess urination. It is cooling and drying in nature, and is considered *tamasic*. It acts as an anti-inflammatory, anti-diarrheal, anti-spasmodic and decongestant. Astringent taste reduces sweat. This taste can be found in green vegetables, teas, nutmeg, asparagus and legumes such as chickpeas. Excessive amounts of astringent taste can induce emotional imbalances such as fear, anxiety, amplified mental chatter, as well as other *vata* imbalances. This taste is least agreeable with *vata* due to its cooling and drying nature. It is more beneficial to *kapha* because it helps reduce congestion and secretions. It is cooling to *pitta*.

Sour, salty and sweet tastes are considered the best tastes for long term tonification or rebuilding of tissue, and are good for reinvigorating the overall mind-body system. Bitter, pungent and astringent tastes have more healing, medicinal properties. We need all six tastes in varying degrees in order to maintain balance. Having the appropriate balance of tastes for your predominant *dosha* is considered *sattvic*. These tastes can be effective at balancing and healing the mind-body system, but in excess, any one of them can actually act as a toxin or poison. The appropriate balance of tastes is found in nature itself, not in processed man-made foods. Most processed food and fast food is focused only on sweet and salty taste. The food industry uses these tastes in unhealthy proportions, even excessively, because they know these flavors will increase sales. Too much of any taste is known to be *tamasic*, clouding the mind, dulling energy and creating inertia. The powers and qualities of the six tastes should not be underestimated, since they can be harnessed in order to optimize your health, weight, energy and vitality.

Focus for Today: Taste alone can have a powerful effect on the mind-body system. Taste can be stimulating, mood enhancing, detoxifying and even medicinal. The *doshas* benefit differently from each of the tastes. The body is programmed to seek a state of balance. It is important to note that when you are craving a specific taste, that your body is seeking to return to balance through that taste. It should also be realized that moods are influenced by taste itself. Begin to notice your moods and energy levels and the foods you crave in order to bring them into balance.

Journal: What are some adjustments you will make in your eating based on your understanding of the effects of the six tastes?

Recipe of the Day:

Try the following recipe which contains each of the six tastes!

Spinach-Strawberry Salad with Strawberry-Basil Vinaigrette

(Serves 4)

4 cups fresh spinach
1 cup organic strawberries
½ cup chopped walnuts
½ small red onion, thinly sliced
½ cup crumbled Gorgonzola (optional)

For the dressing: blend together in blender:

Juice of ½ fresh lemon
1-2 Tbsp red wine vinegar
5 to 6 fresh basil leaves
5 to 6 medium very ripe strawberries for sweetness
¼ cup expeller-pressed solvent-free canola oil
Sea salt and black pepper to taste

Daily Food Journal

Date:_____ Intention for the day:_____ Weight:_____

Water: X off one water for every 8 oz. of water that you drink. This includes lemon waters. During a cleanse you should have at least 3 lemon waters daily.

YOGI PLATE ➔ ¼ Protein ➔ ⟨ ½ Veggies ¼ Whole Grains

| | | Rate your hunger, mood, energy |
| and after meal satisfaction |
| 1=Low | 2=Average | 3=High |

Time	Meal/ Snack	Food/ Beverage	Hungry?	Mood?	Energy?	Satisfied?
	Breakfast					
	Snack					
	Lunch					
	Snack					
	Dinner					
	Snack					

At the end of the day, reflect on how many
servings you had of the following foods/beverages:

Vegetables (Unlimited)	
Whole Grains (Women 1 -3)	
Fruit (Aim for 2)	
Protein (Aim for 3 or more)	

Did I Avoid?	Yes	No	How Much?
Alcohol			
Soft Drinks			
White Sugar			
Artificial Sweeteners			
Processed Food			
Fast Food			

Alert! Use Meat Sparingly
Consume meat no more than 3 times a week!

List your observations and insights for the day. These include successes and behaviors that need attention:
_____
_____
_____
_____
_____

Day 18: Enhancing the Metabolism

At one point or another, almost everyone has blamed their metabolism for their sluggish energy level and inability to lose weight. Often people notice their metabolism just isn't what it used to be. The metabolism, referred to in Ayurveda as *agni* or the internal fire, naturally slows as we age. What is metabolism and how can we enhance it in order to optimize energy levels and weight?

Our base metabolism is the rate at which the body burns energy in the form of calories when the body is at rest. Metabolism varies from person to person. The higher the metabolism, the less fat is stored in the cells, and the lower the metabolism, the more fat is stored. There are two components of metabolism. Anabolism is the energy the body expends in order to create and build up substances it needs such as blood, muscle, skin, hair, bone, cells, secretions, etc. Catabolism is the energy the body expends in order to break foods down and process them for the body to use. Catabolism creates available energy for the muscles to use, or heat for the body to maintain its core temperature. Anabolism and catabolism use approximately 60% of the body's caloric consumption. Body movement accounts for about 40% of the calories burned. There are then two possible avenues through which we can enhance caloric burn: optimizing the metabolic rate, and moving the body more.

In order to maximize metabolic rate, it is necessary to impact the anabolic and catabolic processes in the body. Since anabolism is all about building the body's cells, the more cell building the body is able to do, the stronger the anabolic rate. In Ayurveda, *ranjaka pitta* is the metabolic process of building tissues and blood. Over-exercising or exercising too vigorously actually has an adverse effect on anabolic rate or *ranjaka pitta*. These actually break down bodily tissues. When the body is depleted by expending too much energy on movement, it is not left with sufficient energy for anabolic processes to rebuild components of cells such as proteins and nucleic acids. This is why you may notice that people who over-exercise have unhealthy skin, hair and nails and aren't nearly as "skinny" as you'd think they ought to be. They also end up having little energy left for enjoying life. Not over-exerting, but having a regular and moderate exercise regime best enhances anabolic rate. This is one reason implementing movement like walking and Yoga can be very effective for weight loss.

Anabolic rate is also affected by the failure to take in adequate calories for the body to build and rebuild. When the body receives too few calories, it lowers its metabolic rate to conserve energy. Over-restricting calories does the body no favors when it comes to weight loss. Instead, once again the building of the skin, muscles, hair and nails will be neglected in favor of building the more vital cells in the body. The body will begin to store everything you take in to prevent starvation. You will notice fat stores begin to accumulate in the hips, thighs and abdomen even when eating relatively few calories. Intake of less than 1200-1400 calories a day results in shifting the body into "starvation mode". Metabolic rate slows. Weight-loss will significantly slow as a result, and in starvation mode, the body starts to store fuel just as squirrels store up nuts in the ground for winter. In fact simply eating breakfast has been shown to increase the metabolism by 10%! Eating foods with low or no nutritional value such as processed foods, white breads, crackers, sugary cereals or processed snacks do nothing to boost anabolic rate. These foods do not contain essential nutrients to build anything in the body. These are just empty calories that end up being stored as fat.

Increasing the efficiency of catabolism is a second way to improve base metabolism. Catabolism is the body's process of breaking down food into energy. This process is likened to the process of *panchaka pitta* in Ayurveda in which foods are digested and transformed in the stomach and gastrointestinal tract. The more energy it takes to break down a certain food, the more energy is burned in the catabolic process. Processed foods have already been broken down, there is no fiber, hull or germ to be broken down in the metabolic process, so it takes less energy for the body to process the processed food. The more we challenge our own system to break down foods, the more calories we burn to digest and to metabolize them. This is a fundamental reason why all calories are not created equally. This is why a person can eat the same number of calories of whole foods and lose weight, or eat the caloric equivalent in processed foods and gain weight. Our bodies were created to metabolize natural whole and living foods; God made foods. We were not created to metabolize artificial, processed, genetically modified, artificially preserved and flavored, pesticide-sprayed foods, or any food created in a laboratory. By eating this way we have taken the first step in creating a sluggish metabolism. If God didn't make it, we should think twice about eating it. God made foods were created in mankind's best interest, for our health and well-being. The food industry creates enticing foods in order to fatten its own pockets, and it has done nothing but fatten us in the process. If we can retrain ourselves to eat foods found in nature rather than foods found in boxes, cans and bags, we are also reinvigorating the metabolism. The longer you eat natural foods, the less tempting and appealing processed food becomes. You can completely reset your taste buds and cravings. I know because I've done it myself!

Metabolism Boosters

There are essentially three areas in which we have the ability to boost the metabolism: specific foods and drinks, eating habits themselves, and lifestyle changes.

6 Metabolism-Boosting Foods and Drinks:

1. **Water:** Water is an important and necessary player in metabolism. First, water enables the breakdown of protein and carbohydrates in the body, helping the body to metabolize stored fat. Without sufficient water, metabolism is sluggish. Proper hydration optimizes metabolism. Second, water is critical in the elimination of toxins from the body through sweat, feces and urine. Without sufficient water to flush toxins from the body, the toxins build and are eventually stored in the fat cells, making each fat cell larger in diameter and weight. Furthermore, toxins themselves slow down the metabolism. While the body attempts to process toxins, energy is directed away from metabolic function. A

German study showed that after drinking water, the metabolisms of both men and women increased by 30%. Water also acts as a natural appetite suppressant. If the body's signals of mild thirst go unnoticed, sensations of hunger kick in. Many times we end up eating when all the body needs is a simple glass of water. Often, sensations of thirst are mistaken for hunger. Next time you are feeling hungry, first try to satisfy the craving with water. You may be surprised to find you were not really hungry after all! Aim to drink eight glasses of water a day to optimize metabolism.

2. **Green tea:** Studies have shown that green tea has thermogenic properties. Thermogenesis is the process of burning calories by the body while it digests and assimilates food. In one study, this rate increased by 4% by drinking green tea. Green tea has also been proven to promote fat oxidation. Fat oxidation is the process whereby fat is converted into energy. One study showed that fat oxidation increased 17% after green tea was consumed compared to a placebo. Green tea has also been shown to improve levels of insulin resistance and glucose sensitivity which are often factors in weight gain. Beyond the metabolic properties of green tea, it contains flavonoids, powerful antioxidants, which reduce inflammation, promote heart health, protect cells from damage, prevent some forms of cancer, and protect against Alzheimer's and dementia. With so many benefits, it makes sense to make green tea a regular part of your day. There are some wonderful flavored green teas on the market, which are delicious hot or cold. If you wish to sweeten, use a natural sweetener so as not to undo its healthy benefits.

3. **Heating spices:** Heating spices such as ginger, cinnamon, cardamom, chili peppers, and black pepper are shown to increase core body temperature and promote sweating. Increasing the body's core temperature raises the metabolic rate. Chai tea contains many of these metabolism-benefiting spices.

4. **Apple cider vinegar (organic):** There is nothing magic about apple cider vinegar specifically, however, studies show that the acetic acid in all vinegar regulates glucose metabolism, lowering insulin spikes in the blood stream. Insulin is a powerful hormone which triggers the storage of fat. When too much insulin is available in the bloodstream, it becomes very difficult to lose or even maintain weight. Studies also show a second weight-loss benefit of acetic acid found in vinegar. It has been shown to inhibit the genes which trigger fat storage in the body. In Ayurveda acidic foods are said to increase *agni*, the digestive fire, which in essence is the metabolism. With these benefits it may not be a bad idea to use a bit of apple cider vinegar, or vinegar of any kind, in your cooking. I suggest using it in your own salad dressings or drizzled on a baked potato.

5. **Food containing B-vitamins:** B-vitamins are involved in the breakdown of fat, carbohydrates and protein in the foods we eat. They help act as catalysts in the chemical processes that release energy from food, imparting it to the body. They are essential to the metabolic process and aid in the proper functions of cells. The B-vitamins found in natural food sources are much more effective than the artificially created B-vitamins found in most vitamin supplements. Plentiful sources of natural B-vitamins are leafy greens, green vegetables such as broccoli, eggs, fish, legumes, nuts, whole grains, and dairy.

6. **Grapefruit:** Grapefruit has been known as a weight-loss champion for some time. Science is now backing up the metabolism-boosting benefits of this juicy citrus fruit. One recent study showed that when a group of obese people ate half of a grapefruit with each meal for 12 weeks, participants lost between 4-10 pounds. The reason behind this finding is that grapefruit has been found to significantly lower insulin levels in the blood stream. Insulin is a hormone which tells the body to store fat. Grapefruit is found to lower insulin whether in the form of juice or eating the fruit itself. Red grapefruit contains high levels of the antioxidant lycopene which is known to have anti-tumor properties. Grapefruit can interact with

some prescription medications, so it is important to check with your doctor or pharmacist before adding this fruit to your diet. Personally, I have observed that when I drink a glass of fresh juiced grapefruit with my breakfast, I am less hungry later on in the day. I believe this is due to grapefruit's effect on insulin.

6 Eating Habits Which Affect Metabolism:

1. **Timing is everything:** According to Ayurveda, the timing of eating is paramount. Our digestive fire (metabolism) is the strongest from 10am-2pm, and it is during this time that it is recommended we eat our largest meal of the day. Many cultures around the world eat their largest meal at lunch for this very reason. In fact southern Americans were once known to eat "dinner", their large meal, at lunch, and then a smaller "supper" in the evening. However in modern times with the advent of industrialization, most of America and most of the world eat their largest meals in the evening when the metabolism or *agni* is said to be at its lowest. This results in weight gain and also the accumulation of toxins in the system. When a large meal is eaten while metabolism is at its lowest, digestion is slow and sluggish. Poorly digested food begins to rot in the intestines while we sleep, allowing toxins to accumulate and absorb into the body. We awaken feeling stiff, achy and sluggish.

   Snacking is important and is not forbidden on the Enlightened Eating plan. If you find yourself hungry between meals, then this is a sign that you did not overeat at the last meal. Overeating puts a damper on the digestive fire, over-taxing the system, making the metabolism dull and sluggish and once again resulting in the accumulation of toxins in the intestines. Instead of eating large meals, it is important to eat moderate meals, knowing that it is OK to snack if you are hungry. Snacking does not mean having a sugary treat or convenience food, but instead having something fresh and natural, such as nuts, fruit, carrots, seeds or homemade all-natural treats. Even soup makes a healthful and filling snack! It is important with snacking to note two things. First, are you actually hungry? Make sure you are not bored, stressed, depressed, just thirsty or mindlessly grazing. Do not eat a snack if you do not feel sensations of hunger first. Second, it is important to wait until the previous meal is digested before eating something else. According to Ayurveda, we should wait 3-4 hours after eating a meal before we eat again. This is because it overtaxes the digestive system and slows the digestive fire (metabolism) when we put undigested food on top of partially digested food. This 3-4 hour rule has been really helpful to me in determining if I am truly hungry. It has made me stop in my tracks at the refrigerator many a time and realize that I am standing there not out of hunger, but for other reasons!

2. **Portion size:** Portion sizes have dramatically increased over the decades with the advent of "super-size" meals, and all-you-can-eat buffets. We have lost our sense of what a normal portion actually is! However, our body's ability to process large quantities of food remains as it always has in human evolution! During the time I lived in France, the French people loved to recount their stories of dining out in America! All of them remember being stunned by the huge size of the plates and the piles of food served on them! No wonder Americans are fat they would say! According to Ayurveda, overeating overtaxes the digestive system, and slows the metabolism. Your body becomes slow and lethargic after a large meal because the metabolism has slowed as the system has been overwhelmed by food! If you are tired and sleepy after eating a meal, then it is likely that your portions are too big and that you are overeating. You should not come away from the table feeling sedated! Another rule of thumb is there is no need for seconds of anything! Taking a second helping is doing a favor for your tongue, but does no favors for your body! Starting today, eliminate second helpings of anything! Finally, this is not a new idea, but as the French people observed, our plate size is huge! Eating on a large plate confuses the mind as to what an appropriate portion size is! Today, begin to eat your meal on a salad plate which is more in keeping with the size of a dinner plate in France!

3. **Toxins:** Ayurveda has known for thousands of years that toxins slow the metabolism, weighing it down and making it sluggish. Now modern science has begun to back up this long-held ancient theory. Recent studies have shown that toxins contribute to weight gain in a number of ways. Pesticides sprayed on our foods and industrial pollution found in our drinking water have been found to slow metabolism and contribute to obesity. Numerous chemical toxins reduce thyroid hormone levels and also block thyroid hormone receptor sites. Proper thyroid function is essential to optimal metabolism. Toxins are stored in the fat cells of humans and all living creatures, giving each cell a greater mass index. When we eat any meat, we are eating the toxins stored in the fat cells of the animal. Meat has been proven to contain fourteen times more chemical toxins than plant food. This is because animals are higher up in the food chain and have ingested environmental toxins themselves. Toxins have been shown in studies to decrease the body's ability to burn fat. The liver functions to break down fat and also filter toxins from the body. The more toxins the liver is asked to filter from the body, the less energy it has to expend on breaking down fat, and the more sluggish this process becomes. Although we cannot control all of the toxins we are exposed to in the environment, we can control what we ingest. Avoiding chemical additives, artificial colors, flavors, and preservatives, as well as foods sprayed with pesticides or meats from factory farmed animals will make a tremendous difference in how many toxins the body is exposed to. By simply switching over to primarily organic foods and opting for a vegetarian diet myself, I quickly lost several pounds.

4. **Food temperature:** According to Ayurveda, eating ice cold foods and beverages can cool the *agni* or digestive fire, which is the metabolism. It is not recommended to ingest extremely cold items if you want to optimize the metabolism. Many of us are accustomed to drinking iced beverages with a meal. This actually diminishes the metabolism at a time when we need it most. Switching

to room temperature beverages at meals can give the metabolism the boost it needs. It is also true that cooked foods take less energy to break down than do raw foods. The "fire" or heat in cooking mocks the energy of the digestive fire, doing some of its work before the food even enters the body. Raw foods such as salads require more energy to metabolize than a stir fry for example. By increasing the percentage of raw foods in your diet, you are requiring more of your metabolism.

5. **Alcohol:** According to the Cleveland Clinic newsletter, research shows that alcoholic beverages reduce the body's ability to burn fat by 36%. Alcohol has been shown to stimulate the appetite increasing the chances of overeating, while at the same time slowing metabolism. Alcoholic beverages increase the daily caloric intake by 10% just from booze for even moderate drinkers. Even more alarming is the fact that alcohol is converted to sugar by the body, and raises blood sugar levels. This increased sugar results in the release of insulin, which triggers fat storage. Alcohol also prevents the absorption of some types of B-vitamins into the body. B-vitamins, are players in the metabolic process. Alcohol sabotages weight-loss and promotes weight gain in a variety of ways! To lose weight it is important to limit alcoholic beverages to a minimum.

6. **Blood sugar:** Spikes in blood sugar cause the body to release large amounts of insulin, a blood sugar regulating hormone. Insulin then prompts the body to store excess sugar from the blood stream as fat. Large dips in blood sugar cause fatigue, hunger, mind fogginess, and headaches, causing a dip in overall energy. These dips trigger the body to release the hunger hormones which can lead to overeating, which then leads to spiked insulin levels, and thus fat storage. The release of insulin lowers blood sugar so much that blood sugar levels then dip once again and fatigue and hunger reappear. This can become a vicious cycle of overeating and fat storage for many people. Optimizing the metabolism is dependent upon keeping blood sugar levels within a normal range. Regulating your own blood sugar is possible by monitoring your own body

and your own physical sensations of hunger and fatigue. It is just as imperative not to wait until you are "ravenous" to eat as it is to not eat when you are not actually hungry. It is important not to overeat, which ends up dumping massive amounts of sugar into the blood stream. *What* you are eating is equally impactful on blood sugar. High glycemic foods such as crackers, candy, white pasta, white bread and boxed sugary cereals immediately flood the blood stream with sugar, triggering the release of insulin. "Safe" foods include whole grains, such as brown rice, quinoa, sprouted breads, any vegetable, most fruit, nuts, seeds, and healthy fats such as olive oil, coconut oil, and avocados.

5 Lifestyle Recommendations to Boost Metabolism:

1. **Increase oxygen:** According to Dr. Gabriel Cousens, M.D., and modern Yoga teachings, the oxygen we take in supplies 90% of the fuel for our metabolism, and food only supplies 10%. This supports the ancient Ayurvedic principle that the metabolism is an *agni* or internal fire. Without oxygen, a fire will suffocate, for fire feeds on oxygen. How many of us work slumped at a desk over a computer all day taking in weak, shallow, constricted breaths of air? How many times have we caught ourselves stressed and holding our breath? I know I have! We are hardly fueling the metabolism without sufficient breath. It is important to take as many deep conscious breaths as you can throughout the day in order to feed the internal fire and keep it burning at its optimum.

2. **Increase UV sunlight:** Over the past decade people around the world have been warned to stay out of the sun and away from its "harmful" UV rays. However, these very rays have multiple health benefits such as vitamin D absorption, healing wounds and optimizing the metabolism. Full spectrum sunlight also affects and regulates proper hormonal functioning. Hormones play a critical role in weight and in health according to Dr. Gabriel Cousens, MD. (Cousens, <u>Conscious Eating</u>). People receiving too little sunlight can become tired, sluggish, irritable, sleepy and can develop SAD (Seasonal Affective Disorder). These conditions are hardly the

avenue to weight-loss. Sunlight awakens the natural rhythms in the body, which are essential to metabolism, weight loss and health. According to Ayurveda, the *prana* or "life force energy" from the sun is taken in through the eyes and the skin. Spackling yourself with sunscreen and wearing darkly tinted sunglasses blocks this effect. Too much sun exposure can be harmful to the skin in the form of skin damage which can result in skin cancer, but blocking the UV rays entirely is equally damaging to metabolism and to health. Dr. Gabriel Cousens recommends 40 minutes of sun exposure a day for optimal weight, energy and health. According to him, there are more than 40 different health conditions alleviated by sunlight alone. However, it is best to avoid UV exposure between the peak hours of 10 am-2 pm.

3. **Increase movement:** Another way to invigorate the metabolism is through movement. Forty percent of our daily calories burned occur through ordinary movements. However, it is possible to increase the quantity of movements we make and thereby increasing the number of calories burned. Increase day-to-day movements through regular exercise and just moving the body more. Many experts recommend taking the stairs instead of the elevator, or parking further from the store entrance. Pulling weeds, gardening, walking the dog and even cooking and cleaning are great ways to keep your body moving! Even gentle stretching increases the resting metabolic rate. Be creative and find more ways to move!

4. **Increase muscle:** Muscle burns approximately three times more calories than fat. By increasing your body's muscle to fat ratio you will burn more calories a day even at rest, thus increasing the body's basal metabolic rate. In a resting state, fat burns 2 calories per pound, and muscle burns 5-6 calories per pound. Fat and muscle make up the highest percentage of the body's structure. Yoga is one way to increase muscle mass while increasing overall well being.

5. **Increase Yoga practice:** Regular Yoga practice promotes optimal metabolism. Day 9 was all about Yoga, the metabolism and weight-loss. See Day 9 to learn more about ways Yoga can improve metabolism and help with weight-loss.

Focus for Today: You can impact your metabolism, speeding it up or slowing it down, by the day-to-day choices you make. You do not have to be held prisoner by a slow metabolism; there are numerous ways to rev it up! Today remember to pause and breathe, drink eight glasses of water, refuse second helpings, put your meal on a salad plate, incorporate the metabolism enhancing benefits of raw foods, green tea, grapefruit, warming spices, acetic acid, and B vitamins. Avoid blood sugar highs and lows, alcohol and toxins. Get adequate UV sunlight and get your body moving more!

Journal: What are some metabolism boosting changes you plan to bring into your daily routine? Plan out how you will make these changes.

Recipe of the Day: Enjoy this Kripalu Chai Tea Recipe, and the metabolic benefits of the spices it contains.

Mataji's Chai Tea

(Provided by Sudha Caroline Lundeen from Kripalu Center for Yoga and Health)

Chai Masala Mix: (Use this mix to prepare tea as shown below.)

2 Tbsp ground ginger
1 Tbsp ground black pepper
½ Tbsp cinnamon
½ tsp ground clove
¼ tsp ground cardamom

Suggestion: Make this spice mixture up in larger batches and store in glass jar.

Chai Tea:

2 tsp black tea
1 1/3 cups water
2/3 cup milk
½ tsp Chai Masala Mix
Natural sweetener of choice to taste

In a pan, combine all of the Chai Tea ingredients. Heat to just before boiling. Reduce flame immediately. Allow to sit and brew, then strain and serve. Milk to water ratio can be changed to individual taste. Traditionally whole milk is used in chai, but this is optional as well.

Daily Food Journal

Date:_____ Intention for the day:_____ Weight:_____

Water: ☐☐☐◼◼◼◼◼ *X off one water for every 8 oz. of water that you drink. This includes lemon waters. During a cleanse you should have at least 3 lemon waters daily.*

YOGI PLATE ➡

¼ Protein ─
¼ Whole Grains ─
½ Veggies

Rate your hunger, mood, energy
and after meal satisfaction
1=Low 2=Average 3=High

Time	Meal/ Snack	Food/ Beverage	Hungry?	Mood?	Energy?	Satisfied?
	Breakfast					
	Snack					
	Lunch					
	Snack					
	Dinner					
	Snack					

At the end of the day, reflect on how many servings you had of the following foods/beverages:

Vegetables (Unlimited)	
Whole Grains (Women 1 -3)	
Fruit (Aim for 2)	
Protein (Aim for 3 or more)	

Did I Avoid?	Yes	No	How Much?
Alcohol			
Soft Drinks			
White Sugar			
Artificial Sweeteners			
Processed Food			
Fast Food			

Alert! Use Meat Sparingly

Consume meat no more than 3 times a week!

List your observations and insights for the day. These include successes and behaviors that need attention:

_____
_____
_____
_____
_____

Day 19: *Prana* and Food

"As a culture, we are over-fed, but under-nourished." ~Sudha Caroline Lundeen

In Yoga and Ayurveda, *prana* means life-force energy. It is the same concept as *chi* or *qui* in eastern medicine. *Prana* is that energy that animates the body and gives it life and movement. When *prana* or life-force is ample, no disease can affect us. Disease always involves some deficiency of *prana* in the body. Food also contains *prana* or life-force energy. In Ayurveda, natural whole food is said to be replete with the primal intelligent energy of the cosmos, *prakriti,* which is the basis of all creation. The *prana* in foods is what imparts energy and vitality to us when we eat. Some foods contain high levels of *prana* energy and other foods contain none. Some foods even rob the body of *prana*, leaving you with less energy and feeling more sluggish and lethargic than before you ate. Foods that strip *prana* or life-force from the body include processed foods, fast food, junk food, and foods containing artificial flavors, colors, additives and preservatives.

Since the 50s with the advent of fast food, TV dinners, and convenience food, Americans have become larger and larger. This is no coincidence! These foods are devoid of *prana*, and leave the body seeking energy and craving more food. Once you become in the habit of eating nutrient dense foods you will notice that your appetite and cravings diminish. When your body receives the vitality it needs from food, it is satiated. When it receives none, it continues to hunger for the nutrients it lacks. A person can actually eat large amounts of food and be *prana* and nutrient deficient. For example someone who stocks their freezer with corn-dogs, frozen pizzas, tater tots, chicken nuggets, French toast "stix" and TV dinners, and lives on these foods, is eating a diet devoid of life-force. They may be taking in food, but they are not taking in *prana*, and they are not nourishing the body. This person may even actually be mal-nourished yet over-weight. When the body is filled with "empty" calories, it continues to crave more, seeking needed nourishment.

There are those people who believe that they can make up for their poor diet by taking vitamins. However this is not the case. Most of the vitamins we take are man-made, laboratory created. Studies show that for the most part what we receive through vitamin pills is excreted in the urine. Also, if we attempt to substitute a nourishing diet with a multivitamin, we are not receiving the micronutrients, phytonutrients, antioxidants, fiber, enzymes and trace minerals that are found in plant foods. Scientists are now discovering new nutritional components of natural foods on a regular basis. Also, nutritional science has recently discovered that some vitamins and compounds aren't readily absorbed by the body without the presence of other vitamins and nutrients. Amazingly, whole, natural foods contain these compounds in unison, so that the body is readily able to absorb what it needs from the food. Manufactured vitamins do not fool the body. There is now evidence that taking artificial vitamins may prevent your body from absorbing the much more beneficial natural vitamins and minerals in the foods you eat. Also, studies have recently shown that taking particular supplements can actually shorten life span by increasing likelihood of heart disease and stroke. We need the whole spectrum of nourishing compounds in the right amounts, from real foods in order to live and thrive at our optimal level.

Another reason yet why we should not rely on vitamins: many of the inexpensive vitamins we find in drugstores today are actually manufactured in China. Various contaminants have been found in some brands of vitamins manufactured in China. Also, it has been found that the potency of these vitamins may be quite different from what is listed on the label. The quality control of these vitamins is not reliable.

Prana-containing foods are not man-made foods. Some foods contain higher levels of *prana* than others. The more high-*prana* foods you eat, the more energy and vitality you will have. Foods that contain the highest level of *prana* or life-force energy are foods that are directly from nature. The less processed a food is, the more *prana* it contains. The closer a food is to the vine or the tree the more *prana* it contains. For example, an apple eaten just as it is picked from the tree has more life-force energy than one on the grocery store shelf. An organic apple has more *prana* than a conventionally grown apple. There are two reasons for this. First, it takes more *prana* from your body to process the sprays and toxins found on a conventional apple, thereby stealing back some of the energy it imparts. Secondly, various sources have found that organically grown foods can contain up to 50% more nutrients than conventionally grown foods. We are able to get all of the nutrients we need in just one apple instead of two. We don't continue to hunger or continue to crave, as our bodies have received what they need with fewer calories. By maximizing the nutritional value of our caloric intake through organics, the body needs to take in fewer calories to sustain us nutritionally, resulting in weight loss.

That being said, a non-organic apple from the grocery store has more *prana* in it than commercial apple sauce, because the apple sauce has been further processed. The same holds true for dried apples. Apple sauce and dried apples have more *prana* in them than "apple chips". These have more *prana* in them than does an apple Nutri-grain bar. The apple Nutri-grain bar has more *prana* in it than apple "flavored" cereal like Apple Jacks which doesn't actually even contain apples. The farther the food is from its original form, the less *prana* it contains. Another example would be grains. Once processed into hot cereals or whole-grain breads, they contain less *prana*. When further processed into crackers, cereals or pastas, they contain less *prana* yet. The more processed the less *prana*. The longer food has been away from the vine, the less *prana* it contains. Fresh fruits trucked across the country do not contain the same *prana* as those grown locally. Freshly prepared foods contain more *prana* than left-overs, canned foods, or frozen foods. The "older" the food is, the less *prana* it contains. Foods from the farm, the farmer's market, or fresh from your garden are the highest *prana*-containing foods. Just sprouted foods are said to contain the highest levels of *prana* of all foods!

During my time living in France, like the French, I began doing my grocery shopping every day. The grocery stores are very small, so they get fresh foods delivered daily. The boulangeries or bread stores make their bread twice a day: am for lunch, pm for dinner. The open air markets have the freshest fruits and vegetables one has ever tasted! For the first time in my life I was eating foods at their peak of freshness! I noticed a profound difference in taste, texture and quality over what we find in American grocery stores and supermarkets. It felt like I tasted a real apple for the first time. The strawberries were like luscious, juicy candy at their peak of ripeness, not picked green days before ready and then shipped across country. This is where it really hit home for me how important freshness is when it comes to the flavors and the vitality of foods. These familiar staples tasted nothing like their look-alikes in my home country!

I also remember being dumbfounded when I discovered in France that the restaurants do not dream of providing a take-away box for the left-overs from a meal. The French don't do left-overs! It's no wonder they out-live us, and we out-weigh them! Needless to say, I came back changed in the way I eat.

Our family has begun the tradition of going to a nearby strawberry farm each summer and handpicking our own strawberries. We can't help but eat a few as we pick them off the plant. Until we began this tradition, I have never tasted anything like a strawberry picked ripe and eaten immediately. They are so juicy and flavorful; they seem to have no connection to the strawberries found on the grocery store shelves. After eating a few you can literally feel the *prana* pulsing through your body!

The more life-force energy you get from the foods you eat, the more energy and vitality you will have. After all, our physical body, including the mind, is called the "food-body" or *annamaya kosha* in Ayurveda. There are some natural foods which contain extremely high levels of *prana* or life-force. These foods are called "superfoods". Superfoods are plant foods that contain exceptionally high levels of micronutrients, macronutrients, phytonutrients, antioxidants, and are low in calories. Superfoods are said to have remarkable health benefits, boosting the immune system, fighting disease and slowing the aging process. These foods are said to be particularly effective at managing weight and improving energy levels. These low-calorie, nutrient-dense foods impart the most nourishment calorie for calorie. When your body receives the nutrients it needs, it is satiated on fewer calories, and does not continue to crave more. The more superfoods you manage to work into your diet, the more health, energy and anti-aging benefits you will receive. As the *prana* from these foods pulses through your body, the metabolism is invigorated. The energy these foods impart will have you moving again, increasing your health, energy and vitality. Below you will find a list of high-*prana* "superfoods."

Superfoods

1. Almonds
2. Apples
3. Bananas
4. Beans/legumes
5. Beets
6. Berries
7. Broccoli
8. Butternut squash
9. Dark chocolate
10. Extra-virgin olive oil
11. Flaxseed
12. Garlic
13. Ginger
14. Green tea
15. Kale
16. Organic grapes
17. Pomegranates
18. Pumpkin
19. Pumpkin seeds
20. Spinach
21. Sweet potatoes
22. Swiss chard
23. Tomatoes
24. Walnuts
25. Wheat grass
26. Yogurt (preferably organic Greek yogurt)

Modern society has been through a convenience food phase, a low-fat phase, a low-carb phase and many other phases in between. None of these things have worked. America is fatter than ever and feeling dull and depleted of energy. It is because we are eating foods devoid of life force. How can we expect to derive energy from foods which contain none? It is only when we rediscover the foods that were divinely created to be ideal for our bodies that we will rediscover our ideal weight, and optimal energy, health and vitality.

Focus for Today: When you make your grocery list, make sure it contains high *prana* foods and super-foods! Begin to tune in to your own *prana* or energy as you eat. Begin to notice the changes in your own life-force as you eat nutrient dense foods!

Journal: Tell of an incident in which you became aware of the energy in the food you were eating or the lack thereof. What effects did you notice in your body energetically?

Recipe of the Day:

I always notice a *"prana* boost" from this refreshing drink!

Fresh-Squeezed Lemonade

*I got this idea from the lemonade stand at the farmer's market, but wanted to make it more healthy using agave nectar or raw honey rather than sugar.

1. Squeeze ½ large organic lemon into a tall glass.

2. Place squeezed lemon half into bottom of glass.

3. Add ice cubes to fill glass

4. Fill remainder of glass with water.

5. Stir in desired amount of agave nectar or raw honey.

Enjoy!

Daily Food Journal

Date:_____ Intention for the day:_____ Weight:_____

Water: *X off one water for every 8 oz. of water that you drink. This includes lemon waters. During a cleanse you should have at least 3 lemon waters daily.*

YOGI PLATE ⟶ ¼ Protein ⟶ ← ½ Veggies
¼ Whole Grains ⟶

Rate your hunger, mood, energy
and after meal satisfaction

1=Low   2=Average   3=High

Time	Meal/ Snack	Food/ Beverage	Hungry?	Mood?	Energy?	Satisfied?
	Breakfast					
	Snack					
	Lunch					
	Snack					
	Dinner					
	Snack					

At the end of the day, reflect on how many servings you had of the following foods/beverages:

Vegetables (Unlimited)	
Whole Grains (Women 1 -3)	
Fruit (Aim for 2)	
Protein (Aim for 3 or more)	

Did I Avoid?	Yes	No	How Much?
Alcohol			
Soft Drinks			
White Sugar			
Artificial Sweeteners			
Processed Food			
Fast Food			

Alert! Use Meat Sparingly

Consume meat no more than 3 times a week!

List your observations and insights for the day. These include successes and behaviors that need attention:

_____
_____
_____
_____
_____

Day 20: Optimizing Life-force

In Yoga and Ayurveda life-force energy or *prana* exists in the human body in the same way as energy does in the natural world. It is the energy in our body which animates us and gives us life. When our energy is optimal, it means our life-force is optimal. This life-force or *prana* can be seen through the sparkle in our eyes and the glow in our skin. It is apparent in the way we move, speak, and carry ourselves. We have all known people who seem to have dullness and lack that spark in their eyes. Their movements are heavy and seem to take much effort. Their voice lacks enthusiasm and they lack animation. Something is impairing their life-force or *prana*. I find that I can tell much about someone's life-force simply from the quality of their voice over the phone.

On the other hand, we have all met people who have a certain spark. Their eyes sparkle, their skin glows. They seem to be full of life and enthusiasm. Their movements are light and joyful. Their speech is alive and energetic. Their whole essence is vivacious and effervescent. These are the people we are drawn to. These are people we like to spend time with. These people are pulsing with *prana* or life-force. How can the life-force or *prana* of two human beings be so different?

In nature, in order to create energy, there has to be fuel. Once fuel is present, it can then be burned, which transforms the fuel into energy, which is released. This same process takes place in the body. We take in fuel as food; it is digested or burned by the body and transformed into life-force energy or *prana*. This "alchemical process" which takes place in the body is said in Ayurveda to contain "three vital essences": *ojas*, *tejas* and *prana*. These three essences are responsible for supporting and promoting health in all the bodily systems. What are the vital essences, and what role to they play in our own energy and vitality? How can we optimize our own life-force?

Ojas: *Ojas* is the fuel for the fire in the body. *Ojas* literally means "life sap", and its presence is necessary to fuel the energetic fire or life-force in the body. It can be likened to kindling, whose presence is necessary for the fire to burn. It has also been likened to the oil in a lamp which fuels its radiating light. Without this fuel, no fire is possible. In our body, *ojas* is said to be composed of digested foods, the air we breathe, water, and even the thoughts and impressions taken in by our mind and senses. Without this "life sap", our bodies would be devoid of the fuel necessary to create life-force energy. The quality of our *ojas* is directly related to the quality of the foods we eat, the air we breathe, the water we drink and whether the thoughts and impressions we expose our minds to are uplifting and positive, or heavy and negative. If we put poor quality fuel in our cars, they run for a while, but eventually the engine becomes congested or clogged, and becomes sluggish, and finally the car stops running altogether! The same holds true for the body as well. If you suffer from low energy and a poor immune system, it is likely due to poor quality or depleted *ojas*.

Some of us quickly burn through all of our fuel. We are overworked, over-stressed, overtaxed and exhausted. This leads to "burn-out." If we race a car around all the time revving its engine constantly, we quickly burn through the tank of fuel. If *ojas* is depleted, your lamp cannot burn, your engine cannot run, and the inner fire goes out. Exhaustion sets in, the immune system collapses. Have you depleted your *ojas,* or have you been putting poor quality fuel in your "tank"?

Ojas, our fuel, or "sap of life", is said to be an inner source of calm, patience and sense of well-being. To sustain or increase this vital juice or "primordial soup" in all the tissues, it is important to eat "*sattvic*" whole natural foods that contain life-force. *Ojas* building foods include: organic dairy, almonds, potatoes, sweet potatoes, fresh juicy fruits, cooked vegetables and whole grains. Foods devoid of life force such as processed foods actually deplete *ojas*. It is also important to be mindful of the sensory impressions and thoughts you take in. Negative sensory impressions such as jarring music, violent TV shows or movies, over-stimulation of the senses or negative stimuli of any kind drain *ojas*. Positive thoughts and impressions enhance it.

Tejas: Once sufficient *ojas* or fuel is present, it is then necessary for *tejas* or fire to be there to convert it into energy. *Tejas* is the internal "fire" which transforms the "life sap" or *ojas* into vital life-force. It is the "engine" so to speak which burns the fuel. It is through the energy of *tejas* that digestion takes place. *Tejas* digests not only food, but air, water, thoughts, and sensory impressions as well. As these elements are digested, they are transformed, giving us the energy of life. *Tejas* also relates to our immune system. It is your first line of defense in that it uses its heat energy to burn away and destroy pathogens and toxins. *Tejas* is the fire of a fever. The flames of *tejas* are vital to energy and to health. If our "fire" is not adequate then life-force itself cannot be sufficiently produced. A car may look like it is in perfect condition, but if the engine isn't able to burn the gas, it won't get you anywhere!

Tejas is related to the fire of the metabolism and immune system. It is also said to empower the "fire" of courage, confidence and will-power. It governs the "digestion" of *ojas*, the life giving juices of everything the body takes in. The fire of *tejas* is said to create inner and outer radiance. A weak fire fails to burn and transform these things into energy necessary to create action. Excess *tejas* is just as harmful. It can deplete the stores of *ojas* in the body leading to "burn-out". The quality of the digestive fire in Ayurveda is essential to health and vitality. Too much or too little "fire" can affect overall energy levels. How well is your inner fire functioning?

Yoga and Ayurveda can work to strengthen this fire. Yoga practice and *pranayama* (yogic breath) stimulate *tejas.* Yoga breathing provides the air to fan the flames of *tejas*, increasing the fire. Meditation and concentration increase this fire as well. Allowing food to properly digest also keeps this fire energy fueled. This involves eating foods that are readily digestible, which do not weigh down the digestive fire. Fresh foods, fruits and vegetables, grains, seeds and nuts do not over-tax the digestive fire. Meats, processed and chemically created foods weigh down the system, decreasing the strength of the fire, and lessening the output of *prana* or energy. Iced beverages and eating again before food has had a chance to digest diminish *tejas*. Overeating dampens the digestive fire because a fire needs air and space to burn. Eating right before bed when the digestive fire is at its weakest also decreases *tejas,* smothering the fire further. Any of these actions results in a lower out-put of *prana* energy, and also a reduced metabolism.

Prana: If *ojas* and *tejas* are optimal, then the output of *prana* or life force energy will be ideal, just as a well-built fire burns efficiently with the right fuel and air to support it. When this happens in the body, all systems in the body are provided with the *prana* they need to function and thrive to their highest potential.

Prana is the energy produced through the digestion and transformation of *ojas* or fuel in the body. It is the vital force of life. *Prana* is the energy that supports movement in all bodily systems. It is responsible for enthusiasm, inspiration, and creativity. Without *prana*, we could not walk, talk, work, or play. Without *prana*, the heart would not beat and the lungs would not fill with air. Life would cease to exist. The existence of *prana* is only possible through the presence of sufficient *ojas* and *tejas*. If you find that you are lacking in energy and vitality, then there is a deficiency in the quality of one of these. Low energy is a precursor to disease. It is a signal to your body that something is wrong. It is a signal that either there is not adequate or good quality fuel, or that the inner "fire" is not functioning ideally. When *prana* is optimal, disease cannot exist. Without sufficient *prana*, the body is hospitable to disease. Ayurveda is focused on treating the body before disease can begin. Low *prana* is a sign that swift intervention should occur before disease results.

When *prana* is optimal, the body, mind and spirit can function most efficiently. *Prana* can be increased further through Yoga practice, *pranayama* or Yoga breathing and meditation. However, excess *prana* dries up the juices of *ojas*. Too much *prana* can create restlessness, nervousness, difficulty concentrating and insomnia.

As you can see, each of these three vital elements is dependent on one another. When one of these elements is weak, it weakens the workings of all other elements. If there is insufficient fuel for a fire, the fire burns out. If there is no fire, the fuel is useless. Without these two, energy cannot be created. Excess *tejas* "burns" up *ojas* causing it to become depleted, and the result is mental, physical and spiritual exhaustion. However, excess *ojas* can cause a person to become overly lethargic. Ultimately, it is the right balance of these three which allows us to radiate with energy, vitality, and youthfulness. When we have it, it is obvious by the way we look, feel and move. Yoga and Ayurveda aim to nurture all three of these "vital essences" in order to harmonize the mind-body system. This harmony optimizes your life force.

Focus for Today: Assess your own energy level. How is your immune system? Do you feel vibrant and full of energy and life? Is your life-force at its optimum?

Journal: Are you "burned out"? Has too much *prana*, movement, restlessness, overworking or stress, depleted your stores of "life sap"? Is your inner "fire" burning optimally? How are your stores of *ojas* or fuel? Is it good quality fuel? Is there enough or is it depleted? What lifestyle changes can you make right now to optimize your life-force?

Recipes of the Day:

I find that this soup nourishes the *ojas* in my body. I know it will do the same for you. Enjoy!

Ojas Nourishing Soup

2 15 oz cans organic white bean any kind, drained
6 cloves chopped garlic
1 medium onion, chopped
1 large organic potato, peeled and diced
1 large carrot, diced
3 Tbsp extra virgin olive oil
5-6 cups water or vegetable broth
8 stems fresh Swiss chard, coarsely chopped
Sea salt and pepper

Sauté the garlic, onion, potato and carrot in olive oil. Add the beans and water, simmer for 10 minutes. Add the Swiss chard and wilt. Puree and salt and pepper to taste.

Ojas Nourishing Smoothie

The flavor of almonds and cherries together is divine, and this smoothie is chock-full of life-force!

1 cup cherries with pits removed (the pits contain traces of cyanide)
1/4 cup raw almonds
4 oz water
1 Tbsp agave nectar (or to taste)

Liquefy in blender.

Daily Food Journal

Date:_____ Intention for the day:_____ Weight:_____

Water: *X off one water for every 8 oz. of water that you drink. This includes lemon waters. During a cleanse you should have at least 3 lemon waters daily.*

YOGI PLATE → ¼ Protein → ½ Veggies ← ¼ Whole Grains

	Rate your hunger, mood, energy	
	and after meal satisfaction	
1=Low	2=Average	3=High

Time	Meal/Snack	Food/Beverage	Hungry?	Mood?	Energy?	Satisfied?
	Breakfast					
	Snack					
	Lunch					
	Snack					
	Dinner					
	Snack					

At the end of the day, reflect on how many servings you had of the following foods/beverages:

Vegetables (Unlimited)	
Whole Grains (Women 1 -3)	
Fruit (Aim for 2)	
Protein (Aim for 3 or more)	

Did I Avoid?	Yes	No	How Much?
Alcohol			
Soft Drinks			
White Sugar			
Artificial Sweeteners			
Processed Food			
Fast Food			

Alert! Use Meat Sparingly

Consume meat no more than 3 times a week!

List your observations and insights for the day. These include successes and behaviors that need attention:

_____
_____
_____
_____
_____

Day 21: Self-Care

"You yourself as much as anybody else in the entire universe deserve your love and affection". ~The Buddha

"I wish I could show you when you are lonely or in darkness the astonishing light of your own being." ~Hafiz

Orchids are my favorite flower. I have them all over my home. These tropical flowers are known to be quite fragile and take special care. They need plenty of bright light and sunshine, well-draining soil, regular fertilizer, and just the right amount of water. If they are well cared for they produce the most breath-taking blooms in the plant world. If they are not cared for properly, they may live, but they may never grow a bloom or flourish to their full potential. We ourselves are not so different from orchids. We too need special care to bloom into the most breath-taking, beautiful and thriving versions of ourselves. Much more precious than even the most beautiful flower, human beings require proper self-care to thrive and bloom into their full glory.

Ayurveda and Yoga are fundamentally about self-care. These sciences teach us how to properly care for our mind, body and soul, encouraging us to take the time and effort, to nourish our best self. The only way to achieve optimal weight, health, youthfulness and vitality is through caring and skillful lifestyle choices, and no one can live your life but you. In the western world, it is our proclivity to wait until things are seriously wrong, and then seek the help of a physician in order to "fix" things. Ayurveda and Yoga teach that it is we ourselves who are our own best doctors. Western medicine is already acknowledging that patients themselves have great intuition into their ailments, and about how to go about healing them. We know that the body was intelligently designed to seek its own balance and healing. Ayurveda and Yoga maintain that illness only happens when lifestyle is not in balance with nature and right living.

In modern society, we are always in overdrive. We try to pack so much into our busy schedules that we become over-stimulated and depleted. We have become desensitized to noticing when we need to rest, eat, sleep, use the bathroom, or just take a mental "time out" from work and pressure. When we begin to ignore the natural rhythms of the body, it will eventually "rebel". Ignoring physical urges and sensations leads to imbalance. Imbalance leads to illness. A primary philosophy of Ayurveda is to stay in touch with the natural urgings of our body, mind and spirit. They will never lead us wrong.

It is ultimately what we do for ourselves to maintain or improve our health, energy, weight, and vitality that will pave the way to looking, feeling and living the way we were designed to. In western culture, we often feel guilty for caring for ourselves. Do not mistake self-care for selfishness! Self-care is about giving the time, energy and devotion needed to maintain yourself without cutting corners. It is about doing all that is necessary to achieve and maintain the "you" that you were created to be. Most people would not become ill or overweight or exhausted if they had cared for themselves properly in the first place. In Ayurveda, pathogens aren't seen as the initial source of disease. Disease occurs only after the body has come out of balance and has become hospitable to pathogens. In Ayurvedic thinking, preventing disease is synonymous with caring for the body in a way that keeps it in balance, making it health-friendly rather than a place where disease can flourish. In the western world we tend to wait until things have reached a crisis level, and then seek the outside help of a professional. The truth is our "best self" is in the power of our own hands.

Ayurveda and Yoga remind us that it is we ourselves who are responsible for caring for our own body, mind and spirit, and we do this through making skillful and healthful lifestyle choices. It is often the small things we do that can have the greatest impact on how we look and how we feel. Making healthy and natural food choices, getting needed rest, and slowing down the chaotic pace of our lives is often more powerful than any medicine. There is no substitute for making skillful and informed lifestyle choices that are in harmony with our mental and physical constitution as well as with nature. If we don't give ourselves the time and effort to take care of our body, mind and spirit, we will indeed pay for it later many fold. You owe it to yourself to treat your body, mind and spirit the way they were designed to be treated. You owe it to your loved ones and to the world to be the ideal person you were created to be. However, you cannot expect your mind-body system to function at its optimum if your lifestyle is not optimal. If you put the wrong fuel in a car and then bang it around, run it off the road and refuse to change the oil, you cannot expect the car to run efficiently or last long. Our body-mind system was made to last, but we have to care for it like the prized possession that it is. Most people do not. The health, energy and vitality of the body are entirely dependent upon nourishing and renewing the whole system.

The "three pillars" of self-care are: adequate rest/sleep, eating nourishing foods, and listening to the natural urges and needs of our body. Without these three pillars of support, we cannot achieve well-being, optimal weight, energy, health or vitality. It is the combination of these three aspects of self-care that builds and maintains *ojas*, the "life sap" from which our life-force or *prana* is created. Missing even one of these three pillars of support, like a three legged stool, we will fall. Omitting just one of these pillars curtails the production of vitalizing life-sap or *ojas*, and as it becomes depleted, so do we.

Don't cut corners on sleep and rest. Adequate sleep is critical to self-care. It is also plays a significant role in weight-loss, energy levels, mood, radiance and youthful vitality. If you are denying your body the restorative process of sleep, no matter how well you eat, you will never uncover the optimal you. Studies have shown that lack of sleep itself plays a vital role in weight gain. Human beings require 7-9 hours of sleep per night. When we receive less sleep than this, hormones are affected, particularly two hormones associated with eating and the appetite: "ghrelin" and "leptin." Ghrelin is the hormone which governs the sensations of hunger, signaling us to eat. Our bodies produce more of this hormone when we lack sleep. Most likely this is because when we are deficient in sleep we are also lacking in energy. Food is a primary source of energy for the body.

Leptin is a hormone which governs the sensation of fullness and tells us when to stop eating. When we are short on sleep the body produces less of this hormone. Without this hormone our resolve to control eating is substantially weakened. Lack of sleep also affects food choices. When the body is out of balance, it seeks balance in other ways. When energy reserves are low due to the lack of restorative sleep, the body craves the quick energy of simple carbohydrates, such as sugars or starchy foods. These high calorie foods give a quick burst of energy, then leave the body feeling even more lethargic than before, which inevitably leads to another and another high calorie, quick energy, food craving. According to an article published on the <u>Psychology Today</u> website called "Double your chances of becoming overweight by not sleeping enough" by Dennis Rosen (Jan.31, 2010), a Japanese study showed that sleeping less than 6 hours a night directly correlated with weight gain. The study went on to show that sleeping less than 5 hours a night almost doubled the likelihood of becoming overweight.

Not only does lack of sleep directly affect body weight and energy levels, but it is also shown to compromise the immune system. Lack of sleep robs us of our youthful appearance, leaving the eyes, face and posture looking fatigued. Sleep heals and repairs the body, imparting vitality and radiance. Actors and actresses who appear on camera are highly aware of the essential role sleep plays in their appearance. The statement "I need my beauty sleep." came from Hollywood!

Eating nourishing foods is essential to building up our *ojas* or inner reserves of energy and vitality. Eating foods that contain life-force imparts their life force into us. Foods without life-force tax our body's digestive and detoxification systems and steal vital energies. Without replenishing our inner reserves of life-sap, our body, mind and spirit become depleted.

My friend "Erika" recounted a story about her divorced mother "Evelyn". To Erika's horror, every night for dinner Evelyn makes herself a TV dinner in the microwave and eats it while watching the evening news. When Erika asked her mother why she didn't bother to make herself something more wholesome and nutritious, Evelyn looked her in the eye and stated, "*I don't love myself enough.*" Love yourself enough to feed your mind, body and spirit life-giving foods. Do not eat these foods while being exposed to the negativity that accompanies the evening news. Negative imagery while eating is said to create toxins in the digestive system as we also "digest" bad news. Feed yourself like a mother feeding her child. As a parent, we try to make sure our children receive the vital nutrients they need to thrive and flourish. Why would we do any less for ourselves? Proper self-care includes nurturing yourself with foods. It is about taking the time to lovingly prepare meals as if you were preparing them for the most precious being you know, for it is! It is for you!

Beyond eating and sleeping, self-care includes tuning in to and fulfilling the body's natural urges. According to Ayurveda, suppressing the body's natural urges can have detrimental effects on one's health. Ayurveda recognizes 14 natural urges: sleeping, crying, breathing, coughing, sneezing, belching, yawning, vomiting, eating, drinking, urinating, defecating, ejaculating, and flatulating. Self-care involves satisfying the natural rhythms, urges and needs of the body. How many of these natural urges go unmet in your life?

I have witnessed first-hand the damage that can occur from suppressing a natural urge. My 14 year old daughter suppressed a cough during a test at school for fear of being disruptive. Instead of the force of air going out, the force of the cough went in and actually perforated her lung. Air then began to leak out into the chest cavity. The condition was excruciatingly painful and resulted in an emergency room visit. This is a vivid illustration of the consequences of suppressing a natural urge. Make no mistake; there are consequences physiologically when any natural urge is suppressed. A Zen student once asked his teacher, "Master, what is enlightenment?" The master replied, "When hungry, eat, when tired, sleep." How simple, yet how many of us suppress or ignore our bodies' own natural needs? Many of us do not even take care of our simplest physical needs. How can we blossom into our optimal self if we refuse to meet our most basic needs?

Self-care involves giving back to one's self. If all we do is give of ourselves, and never give back we become depleted. There are a number of ways we can give back to ourselves. It is important to find an outlet such as some form of enjoyable exercise. I highly recommend Yoga, walking, Tai chi, Qigong and meditation. Indulge your senses . . . Take a walk in nature. Relax your muscles with *abhyanga*, Ayurvedic oil self-massage. Unleash your creativity and find a creative outlet, such as writing, singing, playing or listening to music, journaling, drawing or painting, reading, cooking, or whatever it is that brings you creative enjoyment. Throughout each day, take mini "time-outs" just for you. Take a cup of tea, or do something that replenishes your mind, body and spirit. Spend time with yourself, and really get to know and enjoy you. This is not an indulgence, this is a basic need. No guilt allowed!

Love yourself! Make a commitment to self-care. Self-care involves taking the time to rest when tired or sleep when sleepy. Preparing and eating foods that set the intentions for health and vitality are critical as well as drinking plenty of life-nourishing water. Set aside time to exercise and practice Yoga. Demand time to relax, rest and play. Self-care is a lifestyle choice that promotes *sattva*, and optimal health. Take this opportunity to give yourself permission to take time to care for you! Let your self-nourishing eating practice set your intention for all forms of self-care. After all it is eating itself that will affect the most profound changes in your energy, health, weight and vitality. Without three pillars, no structure can stand for long. Adequate sleep/rest, nourishing foods, and honoring what our bodies need are truly the foundation we need to stand on in order to bloom into the magnificent beings we were created to be.

"Self-love, my liege, is not so vile a sin as self-neglecting." ~William Shakespeare, Henry V

Focus for Today: Firmly commit to self-care. Let go of guilt. Let go of the idea that you have to accomplish a certain number of tasks each day. Make yourself and the care of <u>you</u> a priority. Your body, mind and spirit will reflect the radiance of a skillfully chosen lifestyle that includes appropriate rest, nourishing foods, relaxation and renewal.

Journal: What has been holding you back from taking better care of you? What things must you change, lifestyle changes, that will better enable you to reflect the radiance of living harmoniously with nature and your own body-mind system. What benefits can you expect to see in yourself from this? What benefits can others expect to receive from you taking time for self-care?

Recipe of the Day:

Chick Pea, Cherry Tomato and Sunflower Seed Salad with Ginger-Lime Vinaigrette

(Serves 4)

4 cups baby greens
6 oz organic chick peas
½ small red onion, thinly sliced
1 cup cherry tomatoes, chopped into quarters
1 medium cucumber, chopped
¼ cup sunflower seeds

Toss the above ingredients together with Ginger-Lime Vinaigrette below.

Ginger-Lime Vinaigrette:

Juice of 1 large lime or 1 ½ small limes
2 Tbsp solvent-free canola oil
2 Tbsp olive oil
2 cloves garlic
2 large green onions
1 piece of ginger the size of the top phalanx of a finger, peeled
Sea salt and black pepper to taste

Blend the above ingredients until liquefied.

Daily Food Journal

Date:_____ Intention for the day:_____ Weight:_____

Water: ☐☐☐◼◼◼◼◼ X off one water for every 8 oz. of water that you drink. This includes lemon
waters. During a cleanse you should have at least 3 lemon waters daily.

YOGI PLATE ➡

¼ Protein ➡
½ Veggies ⬅
¼ Whole Grains ➡

Rate your hunger, mood, energy
and after meal satisfaction
1=Low   2=Average   3=High

Time	Meal/Snack	Food/Beverage	Hungry?	Mood?	Energy?	Satisfied?
	Breakfast					
	Snack					
	Lunch					
	Snack					
	Dinner					
	Snack					

**At the end of the day, reflect on how many
servings you had of the following foods/beverages:**

Vegetables (Unlimited)	
Whole Grains (Women 1 -3)	
Fruit (Aim for 2)	
Protein (Aim for 3 or more)	

Did I Avoid?	Yes	No	How Much?
Alcohol			
Soft Drinks			
White Sugar			
Artificial Sweeteners			
Processed Food			
Fast Food			

Alert! Use Meat Sparingly

Consume meat no more than 3 times a week!

List your observations and insights for the day. These include successes and behaviors that need attention:
_____
_____
_____
_____
_____

Day 22: Self-Sabotage

"Our deepest fear is not that we are inadequate. Our deepest fear is that we are powerful beyond measure. It is our light, not our darkness that most frightens us. We ask ourselves, who am I to be brilliant, gorgeous, talented, and fabulous? Actually, who are you not to be? You are a child of God. Your playing small does not serve the world. There's nothing enlightened about shrinking so that other people won't feel insecure around you. We are all meant to shine, as children do. We were born to make manifest the glory of God that is within us. It's not just in some of us; it's in everyone. And as we let our own light shine, we unconsciously give other people permission to do the same. As we're liberated from our own fear, our presence automatically liberates others."
~Marianne Williamson

As you begin to enjoy the positive effects of the 40 Day journey, it is important to keep in mind that there may be a temptation to give in, to throw in the towel, and to sabotage the progress you have made. Self-sabotage is a critical pattern that plagues numerous people seeking to look, feel and be their best. Self-sabotage comes from fear: fear of change, fear of the unknown, and fear of success and higher expectations. Self-sabotage is an unconscious way of solving fear and anxiety that arise when it comes to self-improvement. Many of us fear our own greatness, and our own magnificence. We fear unfurling our best self, and the consequences which we perceive to accompany that. Sometimes self-sabotagers subconsciously think they do not deserve better, or are not worthy of a better existence. In other cases, they fear that even their best self may be rejected by others. Perhaps there is fear of the time and energy it will take to live out and maintain one's full potential. Often people feel unprepared to handle the responsibilities of unleashing their true greatness. It isn't unusual for people to begin to panic once they find themselves approaching their goal. Once the realization sets in that their goal is near, they begin to unravel, slipping back into old familiar patterns that do not serve them or their weight, health, energy and vitality.

Somehow, they are not ready for permanent change. This pattern may happen time and time again for a person, until they are able to break out of the pattern of repeated of self-sabotage. In order to overcome self-sabotage, awareness is essential.

Psychologist and Yoga instructor Carolyn Baxter, MD notes that it is familiarity with old habits that brings us a sense of comfort. She says we often confuse familiarity with *comfortable*. Old, unproductive behaviors can seem like an old and faithful friend, and there is a sense of emptiness when that friend is removed from our life. For some, this friend is cigarettes or alcohol, for others it is sugar, sodas, or junk food and the extra weight and lack of vitality which inevitably come along with it.

Dr. Baxter has even encountered this experience first-hand. She recounts how after paying off her student loan from medical school after 11 years of debt, she was shocked to discover a sense of unease having the extra money in her budget. It felt unfamiliar to no longer have the debt hanging over her. She remembers having a very strong urge to make a major purchase on her credit card to in order to feel comfortable again. However, through her practice of Yoga she was able to sit in observance of the need to spend. With awareness, she was able to tolerate the discomfort she felt, and over time the feelings simply subsided. She remains debt free, and that has now become her new normal. Clearly she is grateful she didn't react to the temptation to resolve her feelings of uneasiness with the once comfortable weight of debt by diving back into debt. The same can be said in terms of excess physical weight.

Do you notice as you grow nearer and nearer to your goals, you become increasingly anxious and uncomfortable? Do you notice that when you begin to see great progress in the changes you have made, you suddenly begin to slip and backslide back into your old "comfortable" ways? This self-sabotage pattern happens with recovering alcoholics, gamblers and drug addicts, but it also happens to people who change their patterns of exercise and eating. Once the weight begins to come off, people begin to feel better and more energetic. There are things that one is now physically able to do which might not have been possible before. Some of these things are pleasant, but others are not, such as shoveling snow or cleaning the house. When people begin to look better, they begin to receive compliments and attention. Being unused to this newfound attention, they become uncomfortable. Perhaps members of the opposite sex begin to take interest. Perhaps friends and colleagues become a bit jealous. These experiences can bring on a new sense of unease, and leave us not knowing how to react other than reverting back to old ways of being.

It has even been theorized that the excess girth keeps other people at a distance, acting as an insulation or buffer zone. Perhaps you are uncomfortable with letting people get "close" to you mentally or physically. The new experiences that come along with better health and lower weight are unfamiliar and uncomfortable. In order to move through the initial discomfort of the unknown, it is essential to sit in awareness of the feelings that are surfacing. No need to react, just observe without judgment. As you continue to sit with the feelings that arise, you will notice that they begin to lessen over time. As was the case with Dr. Baxter, eventually the new normal will become familiar and comfortable. In order to pass through the temptation to sabotage your progress, awareness of your fears and sense of dis-ease with a new normal is the first step. Then simply be with the awareness of these feelings, ride the waves of emotion that arise, without reacting. Allow yourself to be in this new space until the unfamiliar becomes the familiar, and the discomfort becomes the new comfortable. This is how we grow and effect permanent change. Perseverance is the path to transformation.

"When I let go of who I am, I become who I might be." ~Lao Tzu

"Great doubt will eventually lead to great change." ~Rabia al-Adawiya

Focus for Today: Take a moment to reflect on the intentions set on Day 3 again. As you near the goal you set at the beginning of the 40 Days, do you notice a sense of discomfort? Begin to sit with any feelings of anxiety and dis-ease that have surfaced as you begin to cultivate a new normal and a new you. Resolve that there is no going back, knowing that as you continue to be with the feelings as they arise, their hold on you will become less and less until the feelings resolve. The new you will in time become the new normal.

Journal: Are you aware of any feelings of uneasiness, discomfort, or anxiety associated with the new you that is emerging? If so, take time to pinpoint what it is you fear about these changes becoming a permanent part of your life. What is it that you fear about becoming your best self? Awareness is the first step on the path to change.

Recipe of the Day:

Pizza is a favorite comfort food loved by all! Pizza doesn't have to "sabotage" your progress! Try these pizza ideas using my own homemade crust!

Elise's Enlightened Pizza

Crust: Makes 1 large pizza

1 cup whole wheat pastry flour
¼ cup ground flaxseeds
1 ¾ cup "double-fiber", unbleached, all-purpose flour
1 tsp sea salt
1 Tbsp extra-virgin olive oil

1 tsp yeast ("quick" yeast if you are in a hurry)
1 Tbsp honey
1 1/8 cups warm water

Mix together the yeast, honey and warm water and let stand for a couple of minutes. Meanwhile, mix the rest of the ingredients together. Add liquid mixture to the flour mixture and knead for 5-10 minutes. I use the dough hook on my Kitchen-Aid mixer to knead. Bread machines are great for kneading or you can knead by hand. Cover dough and allow to rise, 30 minutes. for quick yeast, 1 hour or more for regular yeast.

Pizza ideas: Bake each of these at 450 degrees for 15-20 minutes.

- Top pizza crust with traditional marinara sauce and mozzarella cheese.
- Top crust with sliced roma tomatoes, torn basil, sea salt and pepper, then drizzle with olive oil. Top with fresh mozzarella (optional).
- Top crust with a fine layer of olive oil, minced fresh garlic, sea salt and fresh mozzarella. Optional: delicious topped with arugula tossed in red wine vinegar, olive oil, garlic salt and pepper.
- Top crust with finely sliced vegetables such as zucchini, red bell pepper, onion, garlic, squash or eggplant, and top with Swiss cheese. The vegetables can be pan-sautéed first in a little olive oil and sea salt for a little caramelization if desired.

- Top crust with caramelized onions, sprinkle with sea salt and Swiss cheese.
- Top crust with fresh kale, minced garlic, and cheddar cheese.
- Create your own topping ideas!

Daily Food Journal

Date:_____ Intention for the day:_____ Weight:_____

Water: ☐☐☐▊▊▊▊▊ *X off one water for every 8 oz. of water that you drink. This includes lemon waters. During a cleanse you should have at least 3 lemon waters daily.*

YOGI PLATE ➡ ¼ Protein ⟶ ⟵ ½ Veggies
¼ Whole Grains ⟶

| Rate your hunger, mood, energy |
| and after meal satisfaction |
| 1=Low 2=Average 3=High |

Time	Meal/ Snack	Food/ Beverage	Hungry?	Mood?	Energy?	Satisfied?
	Breakfast					
	Snack					
	Lunch					
	Snack					
	Dinner					
	Snack					

At the end of the day, reflect on how many servings you had of the following foods/beverages:

Vegetables (Unlimited)	
Whole Grains (Women 1 -3)	
Fruit (Aim for 2)	
Protein (Aim for 3 or more)	

Did I Avoid?	Yes	No	How Much?
Alcohol			
Soft Drinks			
White Sugar			
Artificial Sweeteners			
Processed Food			
Fast Food			

| **Alert! Use Meat Sparingly** |
| Consume meat no more than 3 times a week! |

List your observations and insights for the day. These include successes and behaviors that need attention:
_____
_____
_____
_____
_____

Day 23: "Youthing" Instead of Aging!!! The Secrets to Youthfulness, Longevity and Vitality!

"You're never too old to become younger." ~Mae West

For eons mankind has been on the quest for the proverbial "fountain of youth". What if I told you it has been right under our noses all along? What and how we eat not only play a role in our weight and energy, but has a powerful effect on our youthfulness, longevity and vitality. How we move and treat the mind and body also play a primary role in optimizing how youthful we look and feel. Every time I attend a Yoga conference, Yoga teacher training, or have the opportunity to be among a group of regular Yoga practitioners, I never cease to be amazed when I discover the actual ages of the participants. Many times I have been absolutely blown away! I have met many Yoga practitioners who look and act 20 years younger than their actual age! What many people do not realize is that Yoga is more than just stretching, it is a lifestyle.

Many people think Yoga is only for the young and flexible, but it is never too late to begin. Actually, people of all ages and fitness levels can benefit from regular Yoga practice. Yoga keeps the body and mind young in a number of ways. First, it has been shown to keep the joints and spine lubricated and flexible, preventing and easing arthritis. It also lengthens muscles, developing flexibility, which is the key to mobility. It is said that if you practice Yoga, you will still be able to bend over and tie your shoes when you're 80! Balance is another benefit of Yoga practice. Older people tend to fall more easily, as the natural sense of balance decreases. Yoga challenges that, and redevelops a sense of balance. Yoga also strengthens the muscles and bones by supporting your own weight relative to gravity, in different positions and postures. Weight-bearing activities are proven to prevent osteoporosis and build bone density. Weight loss is another benefit of Yoga. It is reported that people who practice Yoga, weigh an average of 15 pounds less than those who don't. By weighing less, your body feels, looks and acts younger!

Yoga also keeps the mind young. It has long been known to reduce the effects of stress and tension. This counteracts the stress hormones which are known to cause high blood pressure, heart disease, and have been linked to Alzheimer's. Learning new things is said to keep the brain youthful. There are approximately 500,000 Yoga poses to learn, perfect, and keep the mind active!

Yoga practice is designed to move toxins out of the body through the pores of the skin in the form of sweat, and through the stimulation of the kidneys, bladder and intestines. Toxins in the body accelerate the effects of aging. The physical practice of Yoga was originally designed to open up energy channels in the body, and remove blockages. In eastern medicine, it has long been thought that disease manifests as a result of the accumulation of "stuck" energy anywhere along the numerous energy meridians in the body. Modern western medicine is now beginning to recognize the credibility of this theory through the recent discovery of evidence of energy flow through the body.

There is much anecdotal evidence of yogis living substantially longer than the average human being. Legend has it that there are yogis living in the Himalayas who are 700-1000 years old! One yogi, purported to have lived for 700 years, was Indian saint and sage Devraha Baba, who died in 1989. Apparently documentation exists in India showing he was alive for at least 250 years. Biblically speaking, Adam, Moses, Abraham, Methuselah and Noah were all purported to have lived for hundreds of years. Perhaps this is actually possible! There are animal species which long outlive humans. Koi, whales and giant tortoises are all capable of living in excess of 200 years.

A great example of Yoga's anti-aging effects is my father, who took up Yoga at my urging in his early 60s. One day he was out in his driveway, talking to a neighbor when he tripped over something. Instead of falling flat on his face, he instantly caught himself with his hands, hovering inches above the cement in "crocodile" pose. His neighbor was astonished, and my dad survived without a bump, bruise, or a broken hip! If you are looking for the "fountain of youth", Yoga comes pretty close!

While Yoga is a huge part of the equation, eating and food also play a vital role in the search for the key to youthfulness, longevity and vitality. Cultures with the highest number of healthy centenarians share in common a similar diet. These cultures eat mostly fresh vegetables and fruits, yogurt, nuts and seeds. Their diets are high in omega 3s, leafy greens, fresh berries, and they drink beverages that are high in antioxidants such as green tea or red wine. Not only do they share in common the things they do eat, but also the things they don't eat. Each of these cultures eats very little meat, sugar or processed food.

In addition, these cultures which experience health and longevity have in common a regular spiritual practice. They do not share the same beliefs or religions, but common to all is taking care of the spirit. They pray, meditate, and attend spiritual services regularly, and contend that their faith is a very important part of their life.

The longest living cultures also share in common an active lifestyle. They walk or bike place to place, and remain active even in their later years. Yoga is a gentle way to keep the body active, supple, lean and fit.

Another simple and completely overlooked antidote to aging is water. Water itself may be one of the most plentiful and uncomplicated secrets to youthful appearance and vitality. Water dilutes and flushes toxins out of the body. Toxins accelerate the aging process by damaging the cells in the body. Water also hydrates the cells of the body including the skin cells and the brain cells. Well-hydrated cells function at their optimal level. Poorly hydrated skin cells are weakened, appearing dry, dull, inflamed and saggy. Water plumps up the skin cells and increases the production of collagen and elastin. Water also increases the flow of blood and oxygen to the skin, causing the skin cells to renew at a faster rate. This promotes a more youthful and radiant complexion and helps keep the skin clear, reducing inflammation. In Ayurveda it has long been known that the body dries out as we age. Modern medical science has begun to concur with this long-held ancient observation. By keeping ourselves well-hydrated, we help keep the body and brain youthful. It has been noted that keeping Alzheimer's patients well-hydrated seems to slow the progression of the disease. Perhaps life-long proper hydration is an ounce of prevention! After all, Alzheimer's is a disease linked to inflammation, and water is the most powerful natural anti-inflammatory on the planet!

We do have some control over how long we live and how well the body ages, as well as how well we maintain youthful radiance, energy and vitality. Lifestyle is the fountain of youth! We cannot discount the powerful effects of the foods we eat, proper hydration, keeping fit and active, and maintaining a regular spiritual practice! Perhaps it is the "small things" that we do in life that really are the magic bullet! I'll let you know when I'm 110!

"Youth has no age." ~Pablo Picasso

Focus for Today: Lifestyle is the secret to youthfulness, longevity and vitality! The proverbial fountain of youth has been right under our noses all along! Take an assessment of your own lifestyle. Are you doing everything you can to promote youthfulness, longevity and vitality?

Journal: What are some lifestyle changes you can make in order to begin "youthing" rather than aging?

Recipe of the Day:

Enjoy this "youthing" version of an American favorite, "the taco".

Veggie Tacos #1

(Makes 8 corn tortilla tacos)

1 zucchini, chopped
1 yellow onion, chopped
½ red bell pepper, chopped
3-4 cloves of garlic, minced
4 cups spinach, stems removed
2-3 Tbsp olive oil
Sea salt and pepper to taste
1 Tbsp taco seasoning
8 corn tortillas (preservative-free, organic if possible)

Sauté the chopped veggies in the olive oil and season with salt, pepper and taco seasoning. Serve inside warm corn tortillas.

Daily Food Journal

Date:_____ Intention for the day:_____ Weight:_____

Water: ☐☐☐◼◼◼◼◼ *X off one water for every 8 oz. of water that you drink. This includes lemon waters. During a cleanse you should have at least 3 lemon waters daily.*

YOGI PLATE ➡

¼ Protein ➡
½ Veggies
¼ Whole Grains ➡

Rate your hunger, mood, energy and after meal satisfaction

1=Low   2=Average   3=High

Time	Meal/Snack	Food/Beverage	Hungry?	Mood?	Energy?	Satisfied?
	Breakfast					
	Snack					
	Lunch					
	Snack					
	Dinner					
	Snack					

At the end of the day, reflect on how many servings you had of the following foods/beverages:

Vegetables (Unlimited)	
Whole Grains (Women 1 -3)	
Fruit (Aim for 2)	
Protein (Aim for 3 or more)	

Did I Avoid?	Yes	No	How Much?
Alcohol			
Soft Drinks			
White Sugar			
Artificial Sweeteners			
Processed Food			
Fast Food			

Alert! Use Meat Sparingly

Consume meat no more than 3 times a week!

List your observations and insights for the day. These include successes and behaviors that need attention:

_____
_____
_____
_____
_____

Phase 2: Eating and the Mind

This phase is all about the mind, eating and food. The "what and how" of eating and food are only the tip of the iceberg when it comes to Enlightened Eating. The mental aspect of eating is where the hugest shift must take place in the journey to Enlightened Eating! During this phase of the journey, you will discover how your mind affects what and how you eat, *and* how what and how you eat affects the mind. Here is where the journey deepens . . . Enjoy!

Day 24: Irrational Fear of Sweet, Salt, Fat, Carbohydrates and Dairy

"As for butter versus margarine, I trust cows more than chemists." ~Joan Gussow

The modern diet industry's fads of the day have had us all on a roller coaster of ever-changing "do's" and "don'ts". This has left us fearful and confused about eating foods that are necessary and important parts of the human diet. Never in human history have we been more afraid of foods that are building blocks of healthy nutrition. From an Ayurvedic standpoint sweet, salt, fat, carbohydrates and dairy in their natural forms are not the enemies that the diet industry has made them out to be, but natural and integral parts of a wholesome diet.

Sweet taste in and of itself is considered a vital component of an Ayurvedic diet. However, in the quest to make things sweeter, cheaper, and with fewer calories, the food industry has manufactured refined "white" sugar, high fructose corn syrup, and any number of artificial sweeteners. It is these non-natural forms of sweetening that we need to be concerned about, and not the entire sweet category. Studies are showing that it is these manufactured forms of sweetness, whether high-caloric or calorie-free, which are at the root of weight gain. A recently published Princeton University Study ("A Sweet Problem: Princeton Researchers Find that High Fructose Corn Syrup Prompts Considerably More Weight Gain" by Hilary Parker <u>News at Princeton</u>, July 7, 2011) directly links high-fructose corn syrup to significant weight gain in rats and "abnormal" increases in body fat, particularly in the abdominal area, in comparison to natural sugar. This study makes it clear that high fructose corn syrup is not a comparable substitute for natural sweeteners as the food industry has claimed. High fructose corn syrup is found in soft drinks, salad dressings, ketchup, yogurt, and many other surprising places!

Calorie-free artificial sweeteners, such as aspartame found in *Nutra-sweet* and *Equal*, saccharin found in *Sweet-n-Low*, and sucralose found in *Splenda*, do not trick the body into losing weight the way they were intended to. In fact, current studies are showing just the opposite to be true! A 2010 study in which rats were fed artificial sweeteners for 14 days found that there were correspondingly "dramatic" increases in appetite and intake of calories. This behavior resulted in substantial weight gain in the rats in just 14 days! Even more intriguing was the fact that the researchers also found strong evidence that the artificial sweeteners had slowed the rats' metabolism. We all know people who drink several diet sodas a day and are constantly struggling with their weight. These people are unknowingly sabotaging their efforts by stimulating their appetite, and lowering their metabolic rate at the same time. Here is a testimony from a friend of mine who gave up her habit of drinking multiple diet sodas a day!

"Here is what I have to say about diet soda: I am 44 years old, currently about 100 pounds overweight, and a lifetime consumer of diet colas. Many days I would drink the equivalent of a 2-liter bottle. Of course since it was diet soda, I felt smug and superior to those who drank "high octane" sugar soda and thought I was making the healthier choice. I never drank water, only soda, and it was my caffeine of choice in the mornings instead of coffee. I knew about the research of the effects of diet soda, but never really wanted to give it up, even though I had tried over the years to kick the habit, but my cravings and the easy, convenient accessibility of soda made it difficult. However, about 2 months ago, I hadn't been to the grocery store in over a week and realized I hadn't had a soda for about a week. I was about to start a new job and thought now would be a good time to NOT get in the habit of having soda around to get me through the day, so I very reluctantly passed the soda aisle at the store. I brought a water bottle with me on my first day of work, stopped at the water cooler and filled it up and haven't looked back since. I was surprised that I really didn't miss the soda that much, but I was stunned at the effect on my appetite. It basically has vanished along with cravings for carbohydrates. All my cravings for anything are gone and the only time I feel starving is when I skip a meal, which says to me "physical need," not "psychological need." I will admit that a busy full-time job has kept my mind away from constant thoughts about food and soda, but it has been an Amazing leap towards making my body healthier. Next step, better food choices!" ~Alicia M.

All sweets are not created equal. It is the man-made sweeteners which have detrimental effects on our health, weight and metabolism.

In Ayurveda, the sweet taste is considered the most nourishing of all the tastes. After all, fruits, berries, sweet vegetables, seeds and nuts are some of the most nutrient-dense of all foods. They were created to entice us with their innate sweetness. Breast milk is inherently sweet in order to encourage infants' intake of optimal nutrition for health and growth. Sweetness itself is not the problem. The source from which the sweetness has been derived is the problem. The media and the diet industry have failed to make this distinction.

In Ayurveda, sweetness in taste is essential in also nourishing "sweetness" in temperament and mood. In an Ayurvedic diet, the sweet taste should always come from a natural source, such as dairy, raw sugar, raw honey, agave nectar, molasses, maple syrup, stevia, fruits, sweet nuts and sweet vegetables. Sweet taste is particularly nourishing for the *vata* and *pitta* constitutions. *Kapha* constitutions may also use natural sweeteners; however they need to use them more sparingly due to their already slower metabolisms and the innate tissue-building qualities found in sweet foods. Sweet taste is considered a tissue builder in Ayurveda, which means it increases tissue mass. This is a key reason children crave sweet things as their bodies are attempting to build and expand the bodily tissues. For this reason as adults it is important to eat this taste in moderation. Personally, I found that slowly reducing the amount of sweeteners I added to foods in small increments did the trick. Now I find many sweetened foods taste overly sweet to me. I do not fear sweet-tasting foods, but I have found a way to enjoy them in moderation, understanding their tissue-increasing nature. We no longer need to fear all sweet things as we have been conditioned to in recent years, but only sweetness coming from artificial sources. However, it is important to note that anything eaten in excess is considered unhealthy in Ayurveda. It is also important to know that if you find yourself constantly craving sweets, it may be that you are seeking to replace the "sweetness" you are lacking in your life with food.

Salt is another dietary staple that has been villainized in recent decades, leading many people to avoid salt like the plague. The truth is, salt is a mineral needed for our body to function optimally. Salt is composed of sodium and chloride (NaCl). Sodium is used by the body to regulate fluid balance and to maintain fluid in the cells. Our bodies are composed of approximately 70% saline water. The sodium in our bodies also helps to conduct and transmit electrical signals from the nerves. Salt helps the body to metabolize insulin and helps with hormone production. Our brains are wired to trigger salt cravings when salt levels become too low. Salt is the most ancient seasoning known to humankind.

In Ayurveda, salt is known to improve digestion, increase heat in the body, produce sweat and clear the pores. It is thought to have a clearing effect on the energy channels. Mentally, it is said to have a sedating and calming effect. That being said, excess salt is contraindicated in Ayurveda as it is in conventional medicine. In excess, salt increases blood pressure, dries out the skin and increases thirst. Salt is also considered a tissue builder and expander in Ayurveda, therefore, in excess it can hinder efforts towards achieving optimal weight.

All salt contains sodium and chloride, but what most people don't realize is that all salt is not created equally. Table salt is mined and then refined and processed to the point that all trace minerals are removed. This processing also increases the ratio of sodium per teaspoon, so that table salt has a higher sodium concentration. Chemical anti-caking agents are added to table salt as well. Mineral and sea salts are left in their natural state and still contain their original trace minerals and are free of chemical agents. Himalayan pink sea salt actually contains 84 trace minerals including iron and iodine. This is what I personally use to season my foods. Besides the lower concentration of sodium and lack of chemical agents, I find the flavor to be milder, lacking the sharpness in taste of table salt.

Even though recent studies have shown no link between decreasing salt intake and improved health, it is important to note that anything in excess in Ayurveda is said to create stagnation and dullness. Different people respond to varying amounts of salt differently; for example people with kidney disease may be unable to flush out excess salt, and people with uncontrolled high blood pressure may be sensitive to the blood increasing properties of salt. Salt actually increases blood in the body thereby increasing the inner pressure on the veins. Salt is not a dangerous villain, but as in all things, moderation is necessary.

Fats have been demonized in recent history as well. As a result, in the 90s decade, fat was extracted from most foods, and avoided like the plague. The word "fat", which is also used to describe someone significantly overweight, seemed to be proof enough that this natural element must be avoided at all costs. The low-fat craze of the 90s decade led to an explosion in obesity rates in this millennium! What nutritional experts have come to realize is that fat is an essential part of our diet. Fat keeps us fuller longer and satiates the appetite. Fat lowers the glycemic index of foods, and slows the rate at which simple carbohydrates and sugars enter into the blood stream, helping to keep blood sugar levels regulated. Fatty acids are essential for brain function, healthy skin, absorption of essential nutrients by the tissues, regular bowel movements, and sustained energy. In addition, fat adds considerably to the taste of foods! Too little fat in the diet is known to decrease energy levels, lead to poor absorption of vitamins and nutrients, affect brain functioning and lead to poor memory, concentration, and mood. Omega 3 fatty acids are known to improve mild to moderate depression, improve ADHD in children, and slow tumor and cancer cell growth. Too little fat can lower HDL (good cholesterol) to unhealthy levels, leading to heart disease.

That being said, not all fats are created equally. Processed "hydrogenated" or "trans fats" were created by the food industry in order to increase the shelf-life of foods thereby increasing industry profits. These fats have been shown to clog arteries by increasing fatty plaque, raise LDL or "bad cholesterol", and increase heart attack risk by 50%. Saturated fats, although they are a bit less insidious than "trans" fats also increase LDL or "bad cholesterol", and raise heart attack risk. These fats are animal fats found primarily in meats, cheese, cream and butter.

Knowing the risks associated with hydrogenated or trans-fats, it is important to note which foods provide the "good" nutritionally necessary fats. Nuts, seeds, fish, avocados, olive oil, sesame oil, flaxseed oil, walnut oil, and soybean oil are safe, healthy sources of beneficial fats.

Carbohydrates are perhaps our most recent enemy in the diet wars. Even I jumped on this wagon for a while. I'm glad I gave it a try myself, because what I noticed when I eliminated carbs was I didn't lose weight. I saw a huge increase in the frequency of migraine headaches,

I felt sluggish, lacked energy and my skin looked the worst I've ever seen it. After 3 or 4 months of this, I realized that "carb counting" was not the way to go! I have a friend who has been counting carbs for years now. This friend has not only gained weight and gotten larger, but her skin has begun to look grayish and dry and has developed many more visible lines than mine, and I am several years older. Her skin looks undernourished. Her hair has also noticeably thinned. It is possible this is due to some other issue, but I suspect it is the high protein, low-carb diet that she follows. After all, the physical body is the "food sheath".

Carbohydrates as a food group have gotten a bad "rap". Carbohydrates are a necessary nutrient providing the body with energy and stamina. They are necessary to healthy functioning of the heart, brain, and nervous system. There are a number of health consequences related to a diet lacking adequate carbohydrates including fatigue, low stamina, difficulty concentrating, depression, kidney stones, vitamin deficiencies, and constipation.

Carbohydrates in and of themselves are not the problem. The real problem is that there has been no differentiation in the diet industry between refined carbohydrates and whole unprocessed carbs. The body does not process refined carbohydrates such as white bread, white rice, pasta, crackers, cookies, sugar, cakes, cereals and candy the same way it processes whole grains, fruits, vegetables and beans/legumes. Refining in the food industry is a process in which chemicals are used to remove the fiber, bran and germ from the whole grain. For example, white rice does not grow white. It is created by placing brown rice through a process in which the fibrous outer bran is removed along with the husk and the germ. The remains are then put through a polishing process. This processing considerably lowers the vitamin and mineral content of the grain as well as the antioxidants and fiber. What is left is mainly the starch. Since the refined carbohydrates have already been processed outside of the body in a factory, there is nothing for the body to do. The sugars or starches enter the system much more quickly than whole food, faster than our bodies were designed to absorb them. They go on to create huge surges in blood sugar levels. The pancreas is forced to quickly release large quantities of insulin into the blood stream to protect the body from the surging blood sugar levels which can cause tissue damage; just ask any diabetic. Over time these sharp rises in blood sugar levels lead to insulin resistance, in which larger and larger amounts of insulin are needed for the cells to respond. Insulin resistance is a key factor in obesity, and is responsible in particular for "belly fat".

The human digestive system was designed to break down the whole grain in its entirety, reaping the benefits of the vitamins, nutrients, fiber and antioxidants therein, and allowing the natural sugars to enter the blood stream slowly and steadily, without creating a big spike in blood sugar levels. Whole foods also take more energy (calories) for the body to break down into sugars, starches and fibers. It is the fiber in these whole foods which keep us feeling full longer. Whole complex carbohydrates include all nuts, seeds, dairy, beans, legumes, fruits, vegetables, and whole grains.

It is much more difficult to over-eat whole grains than their refined and processed Cousens which appear in breads, crackers, cereals, and snack foods. It is strongly suggested that grains are a part of your diet only in their whole and natural form the way they were designed to be eaten. Grains are considered in Ayurveda to be excellent tissue builders. They are great post-operatively or for rebuilding injured or damaged tissue and are useful during pregnancy and convalescence. However, it is recommended to keep your servings of grains to 1-2 servings per day if you are not looking to build extra tissue. All tissues in the body are in constant need of rebuilding, so grains are a necessary part of a healthy diet. However, in large quantity, grains are used to fatten cattle and can do the same to us too. Enlightened Eating participants who are looking to lose weight found it helpful to reduce their daily servings of grains to 1-2 servings a day as suggested in the Daily Food Journal.

Suggested whole grains:

Amaranth
Barley
Brown, black and wild rice
Buckwheat
Bulgur wheat

Corn/popcorn
Farro
Kamut
Millet
Oatmeal (in the form of rolled oats or steel cut oats, not instant oatmeal)
Quinoa
Rye
Spelt
Whole wheat (including whole wheat pasta and whole wheat bread)
Whole wheat couscous

Controversy about dairy products has come in and out of vogue since the latter half of the 20th century. I remember to my dismay when as a child, butter was placed on the "hit" list. Suddenly my mother was buttering our bread with a greasy, flavorless, artificially-colored yellow substance, and I didn't like it! Where was the butter? Years later, we found out we gave up butter only to learn it was the yellow "goo" in the plastic tub that was actually making people sick. I also remember when milk became a scapegoat for all that ails us, and the masses switched to soy milk! This was fine until we found out that most soy is genetically modified and sprayed with all kinds of chemicals along with the fact that it has an estrogenic effect in the body. Then it was back to milk, leaving everyone more confused than ever.

From a Yoga and Ayurvedic standpoint, dairy products are considered excellent wholesome foods. The Indian culture has always placed the cow in high regard as it has provided milk, yogurt, cheese, cream and butter, which are staples in the global diet. The cow is not eaten in India, but revered for providing its milk and milk by-products. In Ayurveda, dairy products are known to nourish all of the tissues including the skin, plasma, brain, marrow, eyes, liver, lungs, stomach and kidneys. Dairy is said to promote longevity, vitality and rejuvenation. *Ghee*, made by heating butter and removing the solids, is considered a powerful elixir and tonic in Ayurveda and is considered the best form of fat for the body. Milk is said to help the nerves, mind and memory, and believed to increase intelligence and strength. Dairy is known to have a calming effect, and warm milk promotes sound sleep.

The problem is that in modern society most milk is no longer the high quality product consumed by ancient yogis. In the past, cows were allowed to roam freely and graze upon grass as nature intended. Today cows are often kept in stalls and given unnatural feeds. Very often these feeds contain animal parts and ground up bone which poorly supports the cow's herbivore digestive system or its innate nutritional needs, which in turn affects the nutritive properties of the milk. The feeds also contain unnatural chemical agents and preservatives. Many cows are given hormones to make them produce ever larger quantities of milk, and these hormones are shown to be secreted in their milk. As the quantity of milk produced increases, the quality of the milk decreases. Most dairy cows are routinely injected with antibiotics in order to make up for the unsanitary conditions in which they are kept, where disease is common. Milk is also pasteurized due to the unsanitary conditions associated with cows being kept in small stalls with urine and feces. It is through these practices that the quality of milk is compromised. Not every dairy farmer employs these practices, but these practices are common and pervasive. Non-organic milk has been shown to contain high levels of pesticides, herbicides, hormones and antibiotics, and considerably decreased levels of nutrients. According to Dr. David Frawley, foremost Ayurvedic expert in the west, the poor practices behind modern dairy farming have significantly compromised the nutritive and nourishing qualities of milk. In his book Conscious Eating, Dr. Gabriel Cousens mentions a study in which a set of calf twins were separated at birth. One was given the mother cow's natural milk, and the second was given pasteurized dairy milk such as is on grocery store shelves. The second calf twin died within 60 days. This same study has been repeated numerous times with very similar results. Clearly nutrition is lacking from the average dairy product found in the dairy case.

It is for this reason that only organic dairy is recommended by current Ayurvedic experts. Organic dairy is more costly. However, I recommend using dairy moderately so a little should go a long way and keep expense down. Amish and French butters and cheeses tend to rely on traditional farming methods in which cattle are able to move and graze freely, and they are not pumped with hormones or antibiotics. These farming methods account for the rich clean flavors of their products, and these products are in line with Ayurvedic dairy recommendations. It is recommended that dairy is used in moderation because even organic milk is shown to contain pesticides and herbicides due to environmental contamination. Also, among its many benefits, dairy is known in Ayurveda to increase tissues and growth, promoting weight and fat gain. It is for this reason that milk is generously fed to babies and children. It is for this very same reason that it is best to keep dairy as more of a condiment for adults, unless they are underweight or convalescent. An example of using dairy as a condiment could be a splash of organic milk in your coffee or tea, or a bit of organic cheese sprinkled on a salad, or a dab of organic butter or *ghee* on toast or bread. Dairy should be consumed particularly sparingly by *kapha* constitutions who are already prone to tissue expansion, excess water retention and excess phlegm which dairy promotes. Dairy itself is not to be demonized, but it is the modern practices used in dairy farming which have diminished many of the beneficial aspects of dairy products.

Looking back over the past several decades, perhaps it has been necessary for society to swing back and forth from one dietary trend or craze to another in order for us to realize that it is only a balanced way of eating, one in harmony with nature the way we were created to eat, that leads to optimal weight, health, energy, and vitality. After all, the body has shown us it can't be tricked into balance and harmony.

Focus for Today: Enlightened Eating is not about banishing any one food group or type from our diets. It is about eating a variety of foods that nourish the body, and eating in harmony with how nature intended. This is the only way to uncover our optimal selves.

Journal: Have you jumped on some of the bandwagons described above? If so what did you notice about your weight, and how you looked and felt?

Recipe of the Day:

Today's recipe contains sweet, salt, fat, dairy and carbs in their optimal form and quantity. I think you will enjoy!

Spinach and Ricotta Omelet

(serves 1)

2 organic eggs
3 Tbsp milk
2 cups fresh spinach
1 clove garlic, minced
2 slices onion
1 Tbsp extra virgin olive oil
3 Tbsp ricotta cheese
Sea salt and pepper to taste

Sautee spinach, garlic and onion in ½ Tbsp olive oil. Season with salt and pepper and set aside. Whisk together eggs and milk. Place remaining ½ Tbsp olive oil in sauté pan. Pour egg mixture into sauté pan and allow to solidify over medium-low heat. Season with sea salt and pepper. Place sautéed vegetables on one half of the egg, and top the vegetables with dollops of ricotta. Carefully fold empty half of omelet over top of cheese and vegetables. Serve and enjoy!

Daily Food Journal

Date:_____ Intention for the day:_____ Weight:_____

Water: ☐☐☐☐▪▪▪▪ *X off one water for every 8 oz. of water that you drink. This includes lemon waters. During a cleanse you should have at least 3 lemon waters daily.*

YOGI PLATE →

¼ Protein →
¼ Whole Grains →
← ½ Veggies

Rate your hunger, mood, energy and after meal satisfaction		
1=Low	2=Average	3=High

Time	Meal/Snack	Food/Beverage	Hungry?	Mood?	Energy?	Satisfied?
	Breakfast					
	Snack					
	Lunch					
	Snack					
	Dinner					
	Snack					

At the end of the day, reflect on how many servings you had of the following foods/beverages:

Vegetables (Unlimited)	
Whole Grains (Women 1 -3)	
Fruit (Aim for 2)	
Protein (Aim for 3 or more)	

Did I Avoid?	Yes	No	How Much?
Alcohol			
Soft Drinks			
White Sugar			
Artificial Sweeteners			
Processed Food			
Fast Food			

Alert! Use Meat Sparingly

Consume meat no more than 3 times a week!

List your observations and insights for the day. These include successes and behaviors that need attention:

_____
_____
_____
_____
_____

Day 25: Eating and Emotions, Emotions and Eating

"Gluttony is an emotional escape, a sign something is eating us."
~Dr. Peter DeVries

Emotional eating . . .

Emotions play the leading role in what and how we eat. I firmly believe emotions play a bigger role in how, why and what we eat than the food itself. I have found myself standing staring into the refrigerator or pantry in search of something to eat immediately after receiving a disturbing email or phone call, or after having a stressful encounter with my husband or kids. I have been standing there staring only to realize that I am not even the least bit hungry. I remember once having a very upsetting confrontation with an acquaintance, and upon returning home I called a friend and began to recount the situation while devouring a bag of tortilla chips. She said, "Elise what are you eating? Put it down, you're just upset." Remarkably, I didn't even realize I was eating until she had pointed it out. It was not about the food, and it was not about hunger. Why did I immediately find myself looking for something to eat after an upsetting situation? I believe people, including me, are eating their emotions, literally chewing them up and swallowing them down, rather than confronting them and facing the discomfort of how they feel. Eating becomes a process of storing the emotions inside, just as excess food is stored in the body as fat. Many people are storing their emotions and carrying them around literally as "excess baggage" in the form of excess weight.

What is eating you . . .

Clinical social worker, and author, Bomar Edmonds, MSW, likens extra weight to a buffer against emotional pain, carrying padding against emotional blows, if you will. He also says the extra weight around the middle is likened to arms around the waist, as people literally "hug" or embrace themselves with food, perhaps because they feel they are not receiving adequate support and love from others. According to Ayurveda, body fat itself gives us a sense of ease and being loved and cared for. It is this sense of comfort that overweight people are often unconsciously seeking through eating and food.

Grace Jull, senior yoga and anatomy instructor at the Kripalu Center for Yoga and Health, notes that the function of the fat cells in the abdominal area is to provide a protective layer around the vital organs. She theorizes that the body may automatically increase abdominal fat in individuals who feel insecure, anxious or fearful as a natural defense mechanism, sensing these emotions as a need for additional physical protection.

The converse is true as well, anorexics starve themselves of food literally mirroring the fact that emotionally they are "starving" for love and acceptance. Mr. Edmonds said that anorexics tend to feel that the physical appearance of their body is all they have to offer, and they feel even that does not measure up. Emotionally, they perceive rejection. Their body image is distorted in direct proportion to their emotional need or perceived rejection, Edmonds says. Theoretically, they are making themselves small because emotionally they feel small and insignificant.

These are two extremes, but clearly from these examples, our emotions impact our perception of eating and food. Emotions affect the average eater more than we are even aware. We eat to celebrate happy times and happy emotions. We eat at parties, we eat at funerals.

Many of us swallow down emotions we are not ready to deal with along with our food. We eat to push down sadness, depression, stress, worry and anxiety, loneliness and even boredom. Perhaps tasty foods help us "stomach" things in life that are difficult to "swallow." Often we are not even aware that this is why we are eating. It dawned on one of my Enlightened Eating students that she overate to swallow down her feelings about her job. She had been unhappy in her job for a long time, and eating made the job a bit more "palatable".

In our fast-paced busy culture I believe food is often used to "nurture" ourselves, when we are not nurturing ourselves in other ways. We use food to smooth things over when we find ourselves over-scheduled, over-worked, and over-stressed. This is why self-care is so critical. When we are not allowing ourselves adequate rest, relaxation, and care, we subconsciously look for ways to make up for it . . . a little treat here and there. However, those little treats add up! Taking care of ourselves properly all along keeps us from using food as a quick emotional fix!

"Not creating delusions is enlightenment." ~Bodhidharma

Letting go. . .

I recently ran into an acquaintance who appeared to have lost a good bit of weight. I commented on how good she looked, and asked what she did to lose the weight. Her response was surprising. She said, "I have always eaten very healthy, but just couldn't seem to lose any weight. Over the last several months, I have really worked on letting go of some things in my past. As I have released these things, the weight just came off on its own! If I had known that that was all it took for me to lose weight, I would have let go a long time ago!"

What are you holding on to? Are there past hurts, resentments, anger or grief that you are storing up somewhere in your body. We often say, "I am carrying the weight of the world on my shoulders right now." Or "I am bearing the weight of sadness or guilt." It is as if we intuitively know that holding on to emotions causes us to hold on in the physical body as well.

One of the five *yamas* or five restraints in the Yoga system is *aparigraha. Aparigraha* can be translated as non-clinging. What are you clinging onto in your life? In Ayurveda clinging, grasping, greed or hoarding are considered characteristics of excess *kapha*. Interestingly, excess *kapha* is also responsible for excess weight. *Kapha* is the heaviest and densest of all the *doshas*, being composed of water and earth. I have a relative who is somewhat of a hoarder. The basement, closets and garage are overflowing with things saved for a rainly day. Not surprisingly, this relative also has issues with being overweight.

Begin to examine your life for those things which need letting go. This may take the form of forgiveness. It may involve allowing tears to flow, releasing pain or grief. It may mean going somewhere safe and just screaming at the top of your lungs, releasing anger stored up for years. It could be writing a letter which you may or may not chose to send. I also find journaling to be a great form of release. Today is the day to begin letting go . . .

Food affects the mood . . .

Just as emotions have the power to affect what and how we eat, and whether we hold on to weight, perhaps unexpectedly, the kinds of foods we eat can affect our emotions, moods and state of mind. The right foods are powerful medicines for the emotions, whereas the wrong foods can create mood swings and emotional imbalance. The science of Ayurveda has noted this connection for thousands of years. Onions, garlic, hot peppers, white sugar, white flour, fried foods and mushrooms are an example of some foods which can stimulate and agitate the mind. For someone who is already agitated these are known to aggravate that condition. Unknowingly these individuals may be provoking emotions such as irritability, aggression, anger, sleeplessness, or hostility. According to the science of Ayurveda, over-eating any food dulls the emotions. Perhaps this is why overeating is so common in our culture. Instead of dealing with life stresses or making lifestyle changes to reduce stress, food is our drug of choice to numb the emotions. Sweet foods are said to cultivate "sweetness" in mood. Those who are craving more sweetness in their life may be more apt to crave sweet foods. Meat, particularly red meat, is known to promote inflammation not only in the body, but it inflames the emotions as well. It has been known to cause agitation, irritability, aggression, and even depression. In fact the Indian army was fed a diet high in meats, in order to cultivate aggressive tendencies in the soldiers in order to prepare them for battle. Gabriel Cousens M.D. cites in his book Conscious Eating, a study done by Steven Scholenthaler, PhD on juvenile delinquents who were being held in custody. When their diet was switched from junk food, meat and sugar, to a diet consisting primarily of fruits and vegetables, there was a 48% decrease in all aspects of violent behavior. Clearly what human beings eat affects emotions, behaviors, and moods.

Foods have powerful emotional effects. One of the most recognized effects participants following the Enlightened Eating program have reported are noticeable feelings of emotional balance and enhanced mood towards the end of the 40 Days. Begin to notice how your own emotions affect when, what and how much you eat. At the same time be sure to note how foods make you feel. What foods are you craving and what emotion are they intended to satisfy? Today we are bringing awareness into how our emotional state influences our eating patterns, and also how the foods we are eating affect our emotional balance.

Focus for Today: Before eating today, pause and take a deep full breath. Relax. Take a moment to notice your emotional tone. Take a moment to notice whether you are actually hungry before you eat. After eating, again take a deep full breath. Observe how you now feel. What if anything has changed? Has the food that you chose affected your mood? Begin to cultivate an awareness of how your emotional state influences your eating habits. Also bring awareness to how the kinds of food you are eating affect your mood, for better or for worse. Keep in mind the effects can be very apparent or quite subtle. Check in for even subtle effects.

Henceforth, when you find yourself in a situation in which you are standing at the pantry, cupboard or refrigerator looking for something to eat, first pause and begin to breathe deeply. Relax, taking a moment to notice your emotional tone. Are you anxious? Bored? Are you sad or depressed? Notice your physical sensations. Are you hungry? Are you tense? Is your heart beating rapidly? Do you physically need to swallow down food, or is there an emotion that you wish to stuff down? Eat only if physical sensations of hunger are present.

Begin to let go . . . With some deep self-observation you can begin to uncover those emotions which weigh you down. Make it your objective to let go and move forward in a lighter state of being . . . Do what it takes to let go. This will not only lighten your weight, but it will ease your soul.

Journal: Journal here about what it is that you may be holding on to emotionally. What do you need to let go? This will take courage and faith, but it can be done. Why not start today?

Try to remember a time or two when you have become aware that you were eating simply as an emotional response. How will next time be different? Try to remember a time when the foods you ate caused a noticeable emotional response, positive or negative. Write about your observations.

Recipe of the Day: Soups are warm and nourishing to the body and soul and give a sense of warmth and comfort emotionally. Try this delicious and nourishing soup.

Butternut Squash Soup

1 large butternut squash, peeled with a potato peeler, seeded, and cubed
1 large yellow onion chopped into large cubes, 1 ½" to 2" or you can substitute 2 chopped leeks for the onions as well
½ head of garlic, peeled
Extra virgin olive oil
Sea salt and pepper
5 cups water or organic vegetable broth
¼ tsp nutmeg
1/3 cup maple syrup
Optional: Sunflower seeds or pumpkin seeds to sprinkle atop the soup!

Toss the first 4 ingredients in olive oil, sea salt, and freshly ground pepper and place in a roasting pan. Roast at 425 to 450 for about 30 minutes, until the edges of the squash and onions brown and caramelize.

Take out of the roasting pan and place in a large soup pot. Add 5 cups of water or vegetable broth. Puree either in a blender or with a hand puree wand. Add nutmeg and maple syrup. Sea salt and pepper to taste! Sprinkle top with toasted sunflower seeds or pumpkin seeds.

A great squash cooking tip from Lorrie R.:

Rinse butternut squash, and place whole squash into crock pot, no need to peel it. Add about ¼ cup water. Let the squash cook all day, and at dinnertime it is ready, peeling and slicing it is super easy! What you don't eat can be placed into a freezer bag and frozen.

Daily Food Journal

Date:_____   Intention for the day:_____   Weight:_____

Water: ☐☐☐■■■■   *X off one water for every 8 oz. of water that you drink. This includes lemon waters. During a cleanse you should have at least 3 lemon waters daily.*

YOGI PLATE →   ¼ Protein →   ← ½ Veggies
¼ Whole Grains →

Rate your hunger, mood, energy and after meal satisfaction		
1=Low	2=Average	3=High

Time	Meal/Snack	Food/Beverage	Hungry?	Mood?	Energy?	Satisfied?
	Breakfast					
	Snack					
	Lunch					
	Snack					
	Dinner					
	Snack					

At the end of the day, reflect on how many servings you had of the following foods/beverages:

Vegetables (Unlimited)	
Whole Grains (Women 1 -3)	
Fruit (Aim for 2)	
Protein (Aim for 3 or more)	

Did I Avoid?	Yes	No	How Much?
Alcohol			
Soft Drinks			
White Sugar			
Artificial Sweeteners			
Processed Food			
Fast Food			

Alert! Use Meat Sparingly

Consume meat no more than 3 times a week!

List your observations and insights for the day. These include successes and behaviors that need attention:
_____
_____
_____
_____
_____

Day 26: The Present Moment

"Taking good care of the present we can even transform the past." ~Thich Nhat Hanh

Have you looked ahead to see what comes next in the Enlightened Eating plan? Are you always fretting about each snack and meal? It is said that all we have is the present moment. The past and the future exist only as thoughts occurring in the present moment. When we spend the present moment ruminating over the past or looking ahead, then the present has been squandered. We often forget that especially when it comes to eating and food. We fret over what we have just eaten and what we are going to eat. When we do too much of this, it is easy to become overwhelmed when it comes to eating well. If we begin to look at each eating experience individually, focusing only on the present meal or snack before us, it becomes easier to make choices that are in line with the intentions we have set for our eating.

Take the Enlightened Eating process one meal or snack at a time, one day at a time. Neither fretting about what you ate at the previous meal, the previous day, or the previous week nor anxiously over-anticipating what will be eaten at the next meal. Make the most enlightened choice you can in the present moment. Let that meal or snack stand alone. Be completely present when you are deciding what to eat and with the choices you are making in the moment. Be present to the level of hunger you are experiencing. Be present to what you are craving in that moment. What is your body asking for? What does your body really need? Be aware that the choices you are making for this meal are the only choices you need to be concerned about in this moment. Make the best choices you can right here, right now. Be present as you are preparing the meal. Let each meal enlighten you, by making enlightened choices for that meal alone. Let each meal individually align with your intentions. Remember all you need to be concerned with is the "now" when it comes to eating and food. Don't look back, don't look forward. Savor and enjoy each bite and meal individually in that moment. If you do this, tension, confusion, and worry drop away, and all that is left is the enjoyment of preparing and eating the fresh wholesome food before you.

Enlightened Eating does require some pre-planning to make good eating choices, but it is most important not to allow anxiety and worry about the next meal to take the joy away from the eating. Planning and fretting are very different. Let go of meals you have already eaten, and do not distress over meals you have yet to eat. Let each meal alone set an intention, and bring awareness to what intention you are setting with what you are placing into your mouth. Enjoy the food before you as you eat it, one meal at a time, and one day at a time. Be present to the eating experience in each moment, and you will be an enlightened eater!

"With the past, I have nothing to do, nor with the future. I live now." ~Ralph Waldo Emerson

Focus for Today: Stay focused on the eating experience at hand. Let the present moment set the intention for how you wish to look or feel.

Journal: What changed today when you began to focus only on the meal at hand?

Recipe of the Day:

Enlightened Greek Salad

(Serves 2)

4 cups organic salad greens
1 tomato, chopped (sliced cherry tomatoes are also delicious)
¼ red onion, thinly sliced
¼ red or green bell pepper, thinly sliced
1 medium cucumber, chopped
12 pitted black olives
1 oz feta cheese, grated with cheese grater

Layer veggies on top of salad greens, top with feta and olives.

The dressing:

Juice of ½ lemon
4 Tbsp extra virgin olive oil
1-2 cloves garlic
½ tsp oregano
Sea salt and pepper to taste

Daily Food Journal

Date:_____ Intention for the day:_____ Weight:_____

Water: ☐☐☐▮▮▮▮▮ *X off one water for every 8 oz. of water that you drink. This includes lemon waters. During a cleanse you should have at least 3 lemon waters daily.*

YOGI PLATE ➡

¼ Protein ➡
½ Veggies
¼ Whole Grains ➡

Rate your hunger, mood, energy
and after meal satisfaction

1=Low　　　2=Average　　　3=High

Time	Meal/Snack	Food/Beverage	Hungry?	Mood?	Energy?	Satisfied?
	Breakfast					
	Snack					
	Lunch					
	Snack					
	Dinner					
	Snack					

At the end of the day, reflect on how many
servings you had of the following foods/beverages:

Vegetables (Unlimited)	
Whole Grains (Women 1 -3)	
Fruit (Aim for 2)	
Protein (Aim for 3 or more)	

Did I Avoid?	Yes	No	How Much?
Alcohol			
Soft Drinks			
White Sugar			
Artificial Sweeteners			
Processed Food			
Fast Food			

Alert! Use Meat Sparingly

Consume meat no more than 3 times a week!

List your observations and insights for the day. These include successes and behaviors that need attention:

_____
_____
_____
_____
_____

Day 27: "The Middle Way"

"For both excessive and insufficient exercise destroy one's strength, and both eating and drinking too much or too little destroy health, whereas the right quantity produces, increases or preserves it. So it is the same with temperance, courage and the other virtues . . . This much then, is clear: in all our conduct it is the mean that is to be commended." ~Aristotle

My grandmother always said "moderation in all things" is the key to life. The ancient wisdom behind Ayuveda also supports this truth. In Ayurveda, it is excess or deficiency which causes disease and disharmony. Harmony and balance create health and vitality. Harmony and balance are found in moderation, or "the middle way."

"The middle way" or moderation, according to the Buddha, is the path to enlightenment. He came to this revelation as he observed a lute player, and realized that if the string of the lute was tuned too tightly, it would break. He also noted that if the string was too flaccid, it would not emit sound. The ideal, he realized, was in the middle, when the string was tightened just enough. This realization led to a key life principle called "the middle way". The middle way is a life lived without extremes. Neither extreme self-denial nor excessive overindulgence leads to a life of harmony and balance. The answer lies in the middle.

The same philosophy applies to eating and food. Extreme diets, such as harsh fasts, severely limiting calories, and eliminating entire food groups such as carbs or fats, almost always backfire. When the eater goes to the extreme, the body is thrown off balance. The body is designed to seek balance, and it will take its own action in order to correct the imbalances forced upon it. Both under-eating and over-indulging push the body into over-correcting. Under-eating will cause the body will hold on to every calorie it receives. It will signal the release of hunger hormones. This will eventually lead to rebound weight gain. Under-eating can lead to deficiencies in the nutrients the body needs, affecting immunity, and the quality and luster of the skin, hair and nails. Under-eating affects the overall energy level as well as the clarity of the mind. Without adequate nutrition, the body becomes sluggish and weak, and the mind becomes slow and unclear. When the mind and body are not functioning at their optimum, the spirit becomes clouded and fragile. Hence, our spiritual connection to the divine can weaken.

Interestingly, over-eating produces results similar to under-eating. Over-eating will cause the body to feel sluggish as it is unable to process a large load of food efficiently. Excessive quantities of food tax the digestive system, and slow it down. Because the food is not processed efficiently, toxins begin to form and accumulate. Accumulated toxins affect the body energetically, as well as in its physical appearance. Toxins are responsible for making the body look and feel puffy and bloated. They detract from the radiance of the skin, hair and nails. Accumulated toxins that are unable to be flushed out are inevitably stored in the fat cells. Over-eating also causes the release of excess amounts of insulin. Insulin is the body's fat storage hormone. The mind is dulled by the heaviness and toxins produced by over-eating. Think food-coma. When the mind and body are sluggish and dull, the spirit cannot be radiant.

For the most part, our modern society has not chosen "the middle way". The affluence we have become accustomed to in the western world has led to over-indulgence, especially when it comes to eating and food. We have a population in which 60% of adults are overweight. We have become addicted to indulging every craving and whim when it comes to food just because we can. Historians believe that it was affluence and over-indulgence that led to the eventual fall of the Roman Empire. This cycle has been a trend in civilizations throughout history, in which a fall is precipitated by a culture of excess. This same pattern manifests itself in the human body as well. It is excess food which precipitates disease such as obesity, heart disease, stroke and diabetes.

The middle way teaches us that the momentary bliss that we get from over-indulging in food or indulging in foods that taste good on the tongue but are not good for the body, is short lived. This is because the result is poor health, undesirable weight, premature aging, clouded thinking, low energy and a weakened spiritual connection. The other side of the coin is true as well. The joy over weight loss that results from extremes is quickly extinguished by hunger pains, weakness, headaches, low energy, dry scaly skin, hair loss, and rebound weight gain. When it comes to the journey to Enlightened Eating, the only path is "the middle way" between self-indulgence and self-denial.

The middle way is also applicable to exercise. Ayurvedic principles emphasize that exercise should never over-strain the body. Extreme forms of exercise or exercising for excessive amounts of time do not benefit the mind, body or spirit. The way you treat your body is the way it will treat you. Pushing the body to extremes when it comes to exercise can result in injury, wear and tear of the joints, cause the body to hold on to every calorie you eat, and result in physical and mental exhaustion. Ayurveda teaches that overly intense exercise produces *ama* or toxins in the body. The build-up of these toxins in the body leads to premature aging, weakened immunity and eventually accumulated toxins lead to disease. Over-exercise is not living in harmony with the body. It is the mind or the will forcibly imposing excess on the body. This is not a harmonious mind-body relationship. It is the mind not being kind to the body. If you are not kind to your body, it will not be kind to you, eventually it will rebel. You are unconsciously setting up an adversarial relationship between the mind and the body, and it is a no-win situation. The body will eventually begin to fail you in one way or another, much to the chagrin of the mind. The body and mind must live in harmony together first, in order for the spirit to thrive. Until we make peace with our bodies, harmony between the mind, body and spirit cannot exist.

Over-exercise will not help you lose weight. I know, I have been there! I gained about 40 pounds while pregnant with my second child. After he was born I was devastated by the body that I was left with. I began to exercise excessively 2 or 3 hours a day, trying to shed the pounds. The weight did not go anywhere. My body held onto the weight that much tighter, expecting to need the stored up calories for the next assault it would receive at the gym! It was when I changed my tactic that I began to lose the weight. After all, the over-exercising clearly wasn't working! It was only when I let go of the idea that the more I exercised, the more weight I'd lose, that the weight began to come off.

I took on a more moderate approach, and once my body began to trust me again, the weight began to shed on its own! Scientific studies show no evidence that by increasing exercise there is any corresponding decrease in weight! We have concluded this all on our own, with the mindset that if a little is good, then more must be better! Evidence shows that the more energy we expend in exercise, the appetite is the only thing that increases correspondingly!

A moderate Yoga practice for an hour a day 4 or 5 days a week will change your body, health and life. Walking is also a great moderate form of exercise. I've done them all! I've been a runner, a spinner, a weight-lifter, and biker. I've done step-aerobics, dance-aerobics, free weights and "nautilus" machines. I've done "power" Yoga, kick-boxing, and everything in between. And I can say that I am at my healthiest weight, the same weight I was when I graduated high school, when I walk briskly and practice moderate-intensity Yoga. I am not someone blessed with an amazing metabolism. I am like everyone else in that way, but I've learned that Grandmother was right, moderation works wonders! I notice moderate exercise doesn't increase my appetite. Aerobics, spinning, weight lifting and running made me hungry enough to chew off my arm! I often ate many more calories than I burned due to the unquenchable hunger I felt after intense exercise! It never worked to help me lose weight, moderation did! Excessive exercising also depletes *prana* or life-force energy, leaving little if any energy available for other enjoyable things in life. Without sufficient *prana*, the mind, body and spirit can't thrive.

On the other side of the coin, not exercising or exercising sporadically is never successful in achieving optimal health, weight, energy and vitality. We've all seen "couch potatoes". They really are like potatoes, in their body's rounded shape, in the poor coloring of their pale, chalky, grayish skin, and in their energy level. Our bodies were created to move, not to sit for hours on end. Exercise is even more critical today because so many people have office jobs. Many of us spend hours a day sitting in front of a computer, and our exercise routine is the only chance our bodies get to move and stretch. This movement circulates vital blood throughout the body. It strengthens muscles (including the heart) and improves bone density. It circulates energy or *prana* through all the energy channels in the body. It helps the body eliminate toxins through sweat and improved digestion. Studies show regular exercise promotes longevity. Moderate exercise has been proven to significantly improve mood and enhance energy levels. The increased blood flow to the skin produces a healthy radiant glow. Moderate exercise benefits the mind, body and spirit on all levels.

The universal truth discovered by the Buddha while observing a lute player clearly applies to both eating and exercise. Moderation or the "middle way" is critical to obtaining your optimal health, weight, energy and vitality. Moderation is the only way to achieve harmony between the mind, body and spirit. Not only is "the middle way" the path to enlightenment, but the path to Enlightened Eating!

Focus for Today: It is moderation the leads to success in all areas of life including eating and exercise. Avoiding extremes is the path to enlightenment and enlightened eating!

Journal: List some ways you have gone to extremes in your eating and exercise regimes. Did this work for you? If you noted that they didn't work, take time to plan a more moderate eating and exercise regime that you believe may be more productive.

Recipe of the Day:

Asparagus has astringent properties, and helps the body flush out excess water weight.

Elise's Fresh Cream of Asparagus Soup

1 ½ lbs asparagus, chopped into 1" pieces
3 or 4 cloves garlic, chopped
1 medium onion, chopped
32 oz box organic vegetable stock
3 Tbsp olive oil
¾ cup milk
½ cup plain Greek yogurt
Juice of ½ lemon
Sea salt to taste
Freshly ground pepper to taste

Sauté asparagus, onion, and garlic in the olive oil until softened. Add vegetable stock. Simmer 15 to 20 minutes. Puree in blender or with hand-held puree wand. Squeeze in lemon. Stir in milk and yogurt. Season with salt and pepper to taste.

Daily Food Journal

Date:_____ Intention for the day:_____ Weight:_____

Water: ☐☐☐◼◼◼◼◼ *X off one water for every 8 oz. of water that you drink. This includes lemon waters. During a cleanse you should have at least 3 lemon waters daily.*

YOGI PLATE ➡

¼ Protein ➡ ← ½ Veggies

¼ Whole Grains ➡

Rate your hunger, mood, energy
and after meal satisfaction
1=Low   2=Average   3=High

Time	Meal/Snack	Food/Beverage	Hungry?	Mood?	Energy?	Satisfied?
	Breakfast					
	Snack					
	Lunch					
	Snack					
	Dinner					
	Snack					

At the end of the day, reflect on how many servings you had of the following foods/beverages:

Vegetables (Unlimited)	
Whole Grains (Women 1 -3)	
Fruit (Aim for 2)	
Protein (Aim for 3 or more)	

Did I Avoid?	Yes	No	How Much?
Alcohol			
Soft Drinks			
White Sugar			
Artificial Sweeteners			
Processed Food			
Fast Food			

> **Alert! Use Meat Sparingly**
>
> Consume meat no more than 3 times a week!

List your observations and insights for the day. These include successes and behaviors that need attention:

_____
_____
_____
_____
_____

Day 28: "Practice and All is Coming"

"I hear and I forget. I see and I remember. I do and I understand." ~Confucious

"Practice and all is coming." These are the words of the late Pattabi Jois, founder of Ashtangha Yoga and world renowned Yoga guru. He was known to repeat these words of encouragement to his students as they became anxious for quick results. These words can also be effectively used as you walk down the path of "Enlightened Eating". Learning something new does not always come easy. It is difficult to break old habits and make way for new and better habits to become engrained. You are re-educating your body as well as your mind to eat in a way that promotes health, youthfulness, optimal weight and vitality. This doesn't happen overnight. Old habits are hard to break. Food addictions are hard to break. As we go through this 40 day process, it is important to understand the concept "Practice and all is coming."

Pattabi Jois was also known to say "Yoga is 99% practice, and 1% everything else." This too can be said of Enlightened Eating. Enlightened Eating is Yoga . . . Yoga of the mouth, Yoga of the body, and Yoga of the mind! Remember Yoga means to "yoke" or unite. The Yoga of eating is about uniting the mind, body and spirit through right eating and natural food, in the way that we were originally designed. It is about uniting our eating practices with the way nature intended, knowing that we ourselves are a part of nature. Yoga takes practice to evolve and develop. This is why we refer to Yoga as a "practice". The more we continue to practice these seemingly "new", yet ancient, eating practices, the more they become a part of our being. The more we practice, the difficult becomes easy, and the easy comes without thought! It took me 7 years of Yoga practice to get into handstand. It seemed almost impossible to me! One day the impossible became a reality, as I balanced upside down on my hands! Now handstand is a breeze . . . It all came with practice.

Educators are aware that there are three stages of learning. First, there is awkward stage where inconsistency and more efforting is required. Second, is the robotic phase in which action become more mechanical. Finally, there is the natural phase, in which actions came naturally and are second nature. Enlightened Eating is a learning practice too. There is great power in practice and repetition even when it comes to eating and food. "Practice and all is coming".

"Enlightenment must come little by little, or else it would overwhelm." ~Idries Shah

Focus for Today: Continue to make the Enlightened Eating concepts a part of your routine, and continue to practice, knowing that with practice, everything will fall into place. "Practice and all is coming."

Journal: What is your biggest obstacle when it comes to Enlightened Eating? In what way can you practice this concept to get to a point where it is "a breeze"?

Recipes of the Day: Try this super easy "ice cream" for an "enlightened desert". These recipes came to me from friend, Yoga instructor and raw food enthusiast Erin Pillman.

Erin's Super-easy Vegan Cinnamon-Banana Ice Cream

Place peeled, very ripe bananas into a zip-lock bag and freeze. Remove frozen bananas, and place in a food processor and blend until smooth. Add a generous amount of cinnamon. (It may be necessary to add a touch of water in some food processors.) Scoop into bowls with ice cream scoop and serve sprinkled with cinnamon.

Erin's Mango Sorbet

Peel and remove mangos from pit. Place fruit into zip-lock bag and freeze. Remove from freezer, and blend in food processor until smooth. Scoop and serve.

Daily Food Journal

Date:_____ Intention for the day:_____ Weight:_____

Water: ⬜⬜⬜⬛⬛⬛⬛⬛ *X off one water for every 8 oz. of water that you drink. This includes lemon waters. During a cleanse you should have at least 3 lemon waters daily.*

YOGI PLATE ➡ ¼ Protein ➡ ½ Veggies
                  ¼ Whole Grains ➡

| | Rate your hunger, mood, energy |
| and after meal satisfaction |
| 1=Low   2=Average   3=High |

Time	Meal/Snack	Food/Beverage	Hungry?	Mood?	Energy?	Satisfied?
	Breakfast					
	Snack					
	Lunch					
	Snack					
	Dinner					
	Snack					

At the end of the day, reflect on how many servings you had of the following foods/beverages:

Vegetables (Unlimited)	
Whole Grains (Women 1 -3)	
Fruit (Aim for 2)	
Protein (Aim for 3 or more)	

Did I Avoid?	Yes	No	How Much?
Alcohol			
Soft Drinks			
White Sugar			
Artificial Sweeteners			
Processed Food			
Fast Food			

| **Alert! Use Meat Sparingly** |
| Consume meat no more than 3 times a week! |

List your observations and insights for the day. These include successes and behaviors that need attention:

_____
_____
_____
_____
_____

Day 29: *Pratyahara*

The <u>Yoga Sutras</u> written nearly two thousand years ago by Patanjali is still a revered text in the teachings of classical Yoga. It is in this text that Patanjali outlines eight limbs or branches of Yoga to be mastered. *Pratyahara* is the fifth of Patanjali's eight limbs of Yoga. This term is most often translated as 'withdrawal from the senses'." For the purposes of Enlightened Eating, we will examine *pratyahara* on the "food" level.

The Sanskrit word *ahara* literally means "food", and the word *prati* means "counter" or "against". In its most literal sense, *pratyahara* means "control of food". In its traditional context, "food" applies to anything the senses, mind or body takes in and "digests". On the food level, it means to gain control over what you are eating or ingesting. It means not letting your senses rule your judgments and choices about what you are eating. From an eating perspective, *pratyahara*, means "withdrawal" from eating foods which aren't nourishing. On all levels, it is about gaining mastery over the senses. It is about letting the intellect take control over lower animal instincts, not letting them guide or rule your choices. *Pratyahara* is a skill that is cultivated by strengthening the "muscles" of the mind to shut out or withdraw from negative influences on the mind-body system, and to consciously turn towards wholesome, healthy living. In the realm of food, it involves employing skill when making eating choices. It is training yourself to make choices that are beneficial to your health, energy and vitality.

In a food sense, *pratyahara* is skillful withdrawal from the wrong foods. It might entail avoiding grocery shopping when you are hungry. At the grocery store, it may mean avoiding the aisles containing junk food, and staying around the periphery of the store where produce, dairy and fresh foods are usually kept. It means avoiding non-nourishing foods which may be a temptation. It means taking proactive measures to withdraw from wrong eating choices. We can avoid eating at restaurants where we know we can't resist the "bottomless" basket of tortilla chips, or the gooey sugar-laden desert. It means proactively choosing to avoid buffets where everyone succumbs to overeating. *Pratyahara* is not overcoming temptation, but it is avoiding situations of temptation altogether. *Pratyahara*, in the eating sense, involves keeping the wrong foods out of your home and the wrong foods out of your body. It is training yourself to avoid the soda machine, and the snack machine. It means intentionally driving past the drive-thru. It is not standing near the snack table at a party, nor standing by the bar. It is turning away from temptation, and walking toward what is right for your mind, body and spirit. The more we walk away from foods which are harmful, the more we strengthen the mental muscles to resist again and again. Dr. David Frawley puts it like this, "The problem is that the senses, like untrained children, have their own will, which is largely instinctual in nature. They tell the mind what to do. If we don't discipline them, they dominate us with their demands." *Pratyahara* is developing a conscious self-discipline to avoid foods that are unbeneficial to our well being. *Pratyahara* is exercise for the mind. The more *pratyahara* is exercised in the context of food, the easier it becomes to circumvent the chatter and demands made by the senses, and the easier it becomes to proactively make skillful eating choices. When it comes to food, *pratyahara*, involves taking control over food, and not letting food have control over you.

Pratyahara involves not only withdrawing the senses from the wrong foods, but turning the senses towards the right foods. In a practical sense, we can begin to substitute better options. For example, a calming tea such as Kava tea is a great substitute for a cocktail. Instead of wine, beer, or soda, substituting sparkling mineral water with a lemon or lime is refreshing. Learn to use honey, stevia, or agave in place of white sugar. Instead of greasy, processed delivery pizza, take time to make your own, crust and all. Instead of a greasy hamburger on a white bun, you might eat a veggie burger on a sprouted grain bun. These are only a few examples, and you will create many great ideas on your own. The point is to turn away from things that weigh down the system, and move towards clean life-giving foods.

"If a person can control his mind, he can find the way to enlightenment, and all wisdom and virtue will naturally come to him." ~Buddha

Focus for Today: Begin to make skillful and proactive choices to better avoid tempting eating situations.

Journal: List some tempting foods and food situations that you have difficulty resisting. Now list ways you can skillfully avoid or "withdraw" from these temptations, so that you do not find yourself in situations where it is too hard to resist.

List some of your own ideas for substitutions for foods that you find tempting, but are not nourishing. List some changes you can make to skillfully direct your eating to better move towards right eating.

Recipe of the Day:

Summer Spritzer

This drink is a refreshing substitute for soda!

8 oz. glass carbonated spring water (such as San Pelligrino)
¼ cup fresh grapefruit juice
1 small wedge of lime squeezed into and then dropped into glass
Sweeten if desired with stevia or agave nectar.

Daily Food Journal

Date:_____ Intention for the day:_____ Weight:_____

Water: ☐☐☐▮▮▮▮ *X off one water for every 8 oz. of water that you drink. This includes lemon waters. During a cleanse you should have at least 3 lemon waters daily.*

YOGI PLATE ➡ ¼ Protein ➡ ⟶ ½ Veggies
¼ Whole Grains ➡

	Rate your hunger, mood, energy		
	and after meal satisfaction		
1=Low	2=Average		3=High

Time	Meal/Snack	Food/Beverage	Hungry?	Mood?	Energy?	Satisfied?
	Breakfast					
	Snack					
	Lunch					
	Snack					
	Dinner					
	Snack					

At the end of the day, reflect on how many servings you had of the following foods/beverages:

Vegetables (Unlimited)	
Whole Grains (Women 1 -3)	
Fruit (Aim for 2)	
Protein (Aim for 3 or more)	

Did I Avoid?	Yes	No	How Much?
Alcohol			
Soft Drinks			
White Sugar			
Artificial Sweeteners			
Processed Food			
Fast Food			

Alert! Use Meat Sparingly

Consume meat no more than 3 times a week!

List your observations and insights for the day. These include successes and behaviors that need attention:

_____
_____
_____
_____
_____

Day 30: Eating with Balance

"The key to keeping balance is knowing when you've lost it." ~Anonymous

If you've practiced Yoga, then you are familiar with balancing poses. They are the poses which require the bones to stack and align, and the body weight to be evenly distributed in order to hold the pose for any length of time. If you've been in a balancing pose, you know what it feels like to be in balance. You also know what it feels like to come out of balance and lose the pose. As difficult as it is to stand on one leg, it is equally challenging to balance eating. Eating in balance however, is a major factor in achieving balanced weight, energy, emotions and mood!

Some people eat very little during the day only to turn around and overeat at night. The result is sluggish energy, grumpy mood and weight gain. Consuming the bulk of the day's calories all at once also weighs down the metabolism or digestive fire, giving it more than it can process. Eating the majority of the calories at night is a double whammy because, according to Ayurveda, this is when the metabolism is burning at its slowest. To make matters worse, because the metabolism and digestive system are not able to process so much food on a slower metabolism, the food begins to putrefy in the intestines creating toxins, which in turn weigh down the metabolism, dull the mind and decrease energy. Toxin build-up in the body causes an inflammatory response which brings about effects such as waking up to low energy, mental dullness, aching joints, and unwanted puffiness and water retention in the morning. Some people call this a food "hangover."

Begin to think of your day as a "balance" or set of scales, in terms of eating and food. If the bulk of your eating is done only at night, your energy and calories are all tipping to one side. I have observed people who eat very carefully and healthfully all week, only to go "hog wild" eating with abandon Friday through Sunday. Again, if your week were placed on a balance scale, the weekend would "tip the scales"! There are also people who do not "drink" during the week only to have six drinks on a Friday night. Again the scales are off balance.

The plate itself can be unbalanced with too many starches and too little green. Perhaps there is mostly meat or protein and too few grains, legumes, vegetables and fruits. Yoga theory teaches that a well-balanced plate is ½ vegetables, ¼ protein and ¼ grain. For some eaters, it is their taste that is unbalanced, eating with an emphasis on sweet or salty foods. Unbalanced eating leads to us taking one step forward and one step back, impeding our progress to optimal weight, health, energy and vitality. Is your eating balanced?

Balance is defined as a state of equilibrium, equipoise, or equal distribution. Balanced eating is eating the right balance of food types and food proportions, balancing the food intake throughout the day and throughout the week. Balanced eating is about avoiding any eating practices which lack symmetry. Balance by definition is about equal distribution when it comes to eating and food. When we feed our body in a balanced way, the energy begins to even out. Sluggishness diminishes, and energy is consistent. Mood and emotional balance are directly affected by imbalanced eating. I notice on days when my husband works straight through lunch, he comes home irritable and cranky. When I fail to eat consistently, my mind becomes foggy, and I become fatigued. If I wait too long to eat, I will end up with a headache. The body needs consistent good quality fuel to run at its optimum.

How often do we shortchange the body by not creating a balanced environment in which it can thrive? For the past year our family has had a fish aquarium. If you under-feed the fish, they die. If you over-feed the fish, they die. In order to keep the fish alive and thriving, balanced feeding is essential. Balanced eating is just as important to human beings! Each time we feed the body in an imbalanced way; it will react and let us know in its own subtle or not so subtle way.

To maintain a balanced metabolism, I encourage eating between meals as long as each eating experience is 3 to 4 hours apart, giving the previous meal time to be digested. I also encourage you to eat something that your body (not your tongue) is craving in a reasonable portion.

These snacks need to be balanced so that they are not all sweet or all salty. These snacks should not be processed but something natural such as fresh or dried fruits, vegetables, nuts or seeds. One of my enlightened eating students, "Carol", actually lost weight by adding a snack and a meal to her day. Carol's eating was not balanced. She would eat breakfast at around 10 am and not eat again until she returned home from work and cooked dinner, which was usually around 9 pm. When she finally ate her evening meal, she was ravenous and would end up over-eating. She was eating the most when her digestive fire or metabolism was at its lowest. Her body was also hoarding every calorie she took in, anticipating the long stretch until the next meal. Carol brought her eating into balance by bringing a nutritious lunch and snack to work with her. She began to keep her body fueled throughout the day. When she got home at night, which was still late, she was able to prepare and eat a healthy and moderate meal. Carol has continued to lose additional weight by adhering to this change even after the 40 Days. What Carol needed was balanced eating!

I have a Yoga instructor friend who read a book and decided she was going to become a "fruititarian", meaning her diet would consist entirely of fruit. This friend struggles with her weight, and I think she thought this was the solution. She is very strong-willed so I did not lecture her that our bodies need essential fats in order for the brain to function properly, and that the body needs protein to rebuild tissue. To me it was clear that eating foods from only one food group was not balanced eating! For months she ate nothing but fruit, and she did not appear to lose weight at all. According to Ayurveda, sweet taste alone is a tissue builder. Babies and children tend to favor sweet tasting foods because their bodies are in the process of growing and expanding. According to Ayurveda, eating excess sweet taste, creates toxins. Eating nothing but fruit is eating an excess of sweet taste. After about 5 months as a "fruititarian" my friend went back to eating normally. It was then that I noticed she appeared to lose weight. Eliminating food groups is not the way to lose weight and it is not balanced eating. When I gave the Atkins diet a try during the low-carb craze, my hair became so thin, fragile and weak, that my hairdresser told me I needed to go get my thyroid checked. My thyroid turned out to be fine. The problem wasn't my thyroid; the problem was I wasn't eating with balance!

Balanced eating is about eating in a way that keeps your *dosha* (Ayurvedic constitution) from slipping out of balance. It is about balancing the right amount of cooked and raw foods throughout the day so that the body can absorb the optimal nutrients. Balanced eating is about never letting yourself go hungry, yet never letting yourself feel "stuffed" and heavy. Balance is ever changing. Just as your body shifts and wavers in order to maintain balance when standing on one foot, balance with food is ever changing. When you begin to fall off the slippery slope back to eating in a way that doesn't serve the mind, body or spirit, finding your way back to right eating takes a sense of balance, and sometimes starting over. Cravings and appetite change with the seasons. Hormones and the monthly cycle cause your body to burn fuel at varying rates, so appetite is variable. Physical activity affects eating and the fuels that your body needs. Stress can create a sense of emotional imbalance. Often, people use food in an attempt to balance moods. It is important not to mindlessly use food to balance stress, but to continue to eat in a balanced way while allowing emotions to rebalance naturally on their own.

A balanced exercise regime is a key part of balanced eating. Intense exercise creates extreme hunger. Very often extreme exercisers end up putting more calories back into their body than they burn off. Because intense physical activity leads to substantially increased appetite, an excessive exercise regimen can actually cause weight gain! Moderate exercise does not seem to affect hunger. Extremes of anything never bring the body into balance!

Eating right for your body in the varying circumstances of day to day life is a continuous balancing act! Personally, I find that my appetite increases during the summer months. I am more active, and need more fuel. The *pitta* or heat of the summer months increases *pitta* in my own system, and *pitta* increases appetite! I notice that mid-cycle and again during menstruation, my appetite is much stronger. I do not let this distress me; instead I eat in a way that rebalances this change, honoring the needs of my body. At times I find myself slipping back into old eating habits in one way or another. Once I become aware of this imbalance, I have to direct myself back to a more enlightened way of eating. There is no all-or-nothing when eating with balance. There is no need to be obsessive and no need to be excessive. That indeed is the secret to balance in eating and in life! When eating comes into balance, you will be amazed at how the scales begin to balance along with mood and energy! When you begin to balance one aspect of your life, you will notice the others follow suit.

"Always is always wrong, and never is never right." ~Swami Venkates

Focus of the Day: Balance. Experiment with balance a bit. Come into tree pose. Notice how the mind, body, bones and muscles must continuously shift, move, and refocus in order for you to stay balanced in the pose. When you fall out of balance what do you do? Do you give up or do you try again! This pose can give you so much insight into having a balanced approach to eating.

Journal: Note ways that your eating is currently or has been in or out of balance. What side effects do you experience from imbalanced eating? List some ways you can bring your own eating into balance.

Recipe of the Day:

Super Easy Enlightened Snack

*This snack is a great way to balance sweet and salty taste, and to keep your energy levels balanced!

2 Tbsp olive oil
1/3 cup of the nut or seed of your choice (sesame, cashew, almond, sunflower)
¼ cup honey, molasses or maple syrup
1 teaspoon balsamic vinegar
Sea salt to taste

In a pan, warm the olive oil, add the nuts and sauté them for a few minutes. Add the honey and stir. Allow it to bubble for several minutes, add balsamic vinegar and salt. Bubble a couple more minutes. Pour onto wax paper, or aluminum foil and cool in refrigerator or freezer to speed up the process. Break off into pieces like peanut brittle.

This is great on salads too!

Daily Food Journal

Date:_____   Intention for the day:_____   Weight:_____

Water: ☐☐☐◼◼◼◼◼ *X off one water for every 8 oz. of water that you drink. This includes lemon waters. During a cleanse you should have at least 3 lemon waters daily.*

YOGI PLATE ➡ ¼ Protein ➡ / ⬅ ½ Veggies
¼ Whole Grains ➡

Rate your hunger, mood, energy
and after meal satisfaction
1=Low   2=Average   3=High

Time	Meal/ Snack	Food/ Beverage	Hungry?	Mood?	Energy?	Satisfied?
	Breakfast					
	Snack					
	Lunch					
	Snack					
	Dinner					
	Snack					

At the end of the day, reflect on how many
servings you had of the following foods/beverages:

Vegetables (Unlimited)	
Whole Grains (Women 1 -3)	
Fruit (Aim for 2)	
Protein (Aim for 3 or more)	

Did I Avoid?	Yes	No	How Much?
Alcohol			
Soft Drinks			
White Sugar			
Artificial Sweeteners			
Processed Food			
Fast Food			

Alert! Use Meat Sparingly

Consume meat no more than 3 times a week!

List your observations and insights for the day. These include successes and behaviors that need attention:
_____
_____
_____
_____
_____

Day 31: Eating with Witness Consciousness

"By simply being a witness you are at the highest peak of consciousness, and when you are at the highest peak of consciousness, from there you can look at the deepest depth of your being." ~Osho

"Witness consciousness" is the name given to the practice of watching yourself as a passive non-judgmental observer. It is a powerful tool for self-understanding and self-growth. We each have the unique ability to observe ourselves and our own actions and reactions while they occur without passing judgment. Witness consciousness is often likened to a mirror. A mirror only reflects things as they are. It reflects them accurately, yet does not make judgments. Witness consciousness is compassionate. Witness consciousness is a part of your own inner awareness that you can cultivate by allowing yourself to become a "watcher" of your own sensations, reactions, thoughts and feelings. It is not about thinking the thoughts or doing the actions, but watching yourself as you think them and as you do them, as though you were watching yourself in a mirror.

It is important as you move towards a path of Enlightened Eating to develop a witness consciousness when it comes to eating and food. Begin to passively observe your behaviors, thoughts, sensations, urges, patterns and cravings when it comes to eating and food. Notice and honor the natural rhythms of your hunger. Do this without judgment, without guilt, and honor the needs of your body by feeding it adequately and nourishing it with the appropriate foods. Notice days and times of day as well as seasons when you are hungrier than others.

On the occasion when I do grab something that wasn't such a good choice, I simply observe, without judgment or beating myself up. I make a note to myself to make a better choice next time the occasion arises. I also observe the effects of my poor eating choice. How do I feel energetically? Did this food really satiate me? How does my digestive system feel? Is my mind foggy or sluggish? Did my joints begin to ache? Did it cause a headache? Do I feel energized after eating, or lethargic?

By cultivating the ability to observe your eating as a witness, instead of immediately becoming your worst critic and berating yourself, you are able to develop your own sense of wisdom about eating and food. Conscious awareness gives us the opportunity to intelligently act, instead of reacting. You observe the cause and effect in your eating habits. As you observe how and why you eat and how you feel, you become better able to make informed and conscious choices when it comes to eating. There is no need to panic, no need to judge, no need for chastisement. Simply become an objective witness of your own eating. Cultivating this habit can help put negativity behind us. Witness consciousness is a way of keeping the mind in harmony with our body rather than at odds with it. By observing with non-judgmental acceptance, eating and food are no longer a war. The struggle is gone. Once the struggle is removed, peace and acceptance between the mind and body set in. The mind and the body are one. The essence of Yoga is to unite. Kripalu Yoga emphasizes "self-observation without judgment". It employs the awareness focusing technique of "BRFWA" - "Breathe, Relax, Feel, Watch, and Allow" - as the framework from which witnessing and learning takes place. In order to develop your own witness consciousness, give the "BRFWA" technique below a try:

Breathe-Although the breath is natural and automatic, we often hold the breath or take only shallow breaths. When we breathe in, we breathe in life-force. When we breathe out, we let go and relax. The exhale is the ultimate letting go.

Relax-Once we begin to breathe, then we can begin to relax. As we relax the body, the mind will follow. Once the mind relaxes, it is no longer defensive, and is open and ready to learn.

Feel-Once you have relaxed you can begin to feel. Feel the sensations present in the body. Notice the feeling tone, mood and emotions that are present in the mind. Are you actually feeling hungry? What kind of food is your body really asking for? How did you feel during and after eating? Do you feel satiated, or are you still hungering?

Watch-As you feel the emotions and sensations you are experiencing, then you can observe how you respond to them. From this perspective too you can choose to simply observe the sensations and emotions you are having without reacting. As the watcher, you can simply perceive, and not react. Self-observation is a powerful practice to bring about awareness of deep-seated patterns and unconscious conditioning when it comes to life and to eating and food.

Allow-Allow yourself to just be with the sensations you have perceived. If you choose to respond, allow your response to be natural and unhindered. Allow yourself to be as you are without judgment.

Employ this technique when it comes to eating and food, and you will develop a conscious awareness of what, why and how you eat. This awareness will help you make skillful changes, and also help you stop the war between the mind and body when it comes to eating and food.

"Growth allows a portion of the mind to remain an objective witness even in the face of disturbance. This witness is always there, if one can keep a wakeful attitude." ~Swami Kripalu

Focus for Today: As you encounter eating and food today, consciously approach it as a compassionate observer. Watch yourself and how, when, and why you approach food. Observe how you feel, before, during and after eating. Try the BRFWA technique as you are witnessing yourself without judgment: "Breathe, Relax, Feel, Watch, and Allow."

Journal: Record your observations today when eating. Do not make any judgments, simply record what you noticed and observed just as it transpired. Record your observations, thoughts, feelings and sensations which arose today as you encountered eating and food.

Recipe of the Day:

Blueberry Scones

½ c organic half and half
1 5.3 oz container vanilla Greek yogurt
2 tsp baking powder
1 stick organic butter or *ghee*
1 c whole wheat pastry flour
1 c unbleached all-purpose double fiber flour
1 c rolled oats
1 ½ c blueberries (frozen, fresh, or dried)
5 Tbsp raw sugar
¾ tsp salt
2 tsp vanilla
Extra raw sugar to top scone

Preheat oven to 425 degrees F. Stir together all dry ingredients except blueberries. Whisk together all wet ingredients. Add blueberries to dry ingredients carefully. Fold in wet ingredients very carefully as to not mush blueberries.

Form into oval shaped balls and flatten slightly with hands. Press the tops into the extra raw sugar, and place on a baking sheet. Bake 20-25 minutes, then remove from sheet quickly and carefully and place on a cooling rack. Enjoy!

Daily Food Journal

Date:_____ Intention for the day:_____ Weight:_____

Water: ☐☐☐⬛⬛⬛⬛⬛ *X off one water for every 8 oz. of water that you drink. This includes lemon waters. During a cleanse you should have at least 3 lemon waters daily.*

YOGI PLATE ➡

¼ Protein ➡
½ Veggies ⬅
¼ Whole Grains ➡

	Rate your hunger, mood, energy
	and after meal satisfaction
1=Low 2=Average 3=High	

Time	Meal/Snack	Food/Beverage	Hungry?	Mood?	Energy?	Satisfied?
	Breakfast					
	Snack					
	Lunch					
	Snack					
	Dinner					
	Snack					

At the end of the day, reflect on how many
servings you had of the following foods/beverages:

Vegetables (Unlimited)	
Whole Grains (Women 1 -3)	
Fruit (Aim for 2)	
Protein (Aim for 3 or more)	

Did I Avoid?	Yes	No	How Much?
Alcohol			
Soft Drinks			
White Sugar			
Artificial Sweeteners			
Processed Food			
Fast Food			

> **Alert! Use Meat Sparingly**
>
> Consume meat no more than 3 times a week!

List your observations and insights for the day. These include successes and behaviors that need attention:
_____
_____
_____
_____
_____

Day 32: Eating Mindfully

"To eat is a necessity, but to eat intelligently is an art." ~La Rochefoucald

Mindfulness can be described as attentive awareness in the present moment. It is paying attention on purpose to what is at hand right now. It is staying in tune and engaged with the here and now objectively. This thoughtful awareness should be brought into all things we do in each and every moment, but how often do we forget to bring mindfulness into the simple act of eating? How many of us eat at the computer, in front of the TV or in the car, never being fully present to the colors, flavors, textures, or tastes in each bite? Even more importantly, how little attention do we give to how well we chew our food or how much we are eating? Do we even pay attention to whether we are really hungry? Do we keep eating without noticing when we are actually full? Eating mindfully involves awareness of the entire eating process from beginning to finish. Have you ever caught yourself eating and didn't even realize you were eating? Have you ever begun eating and continued to do so until you realized you had eaten the whole bag of chips or the whole sleeve of cookies?

What eating mindfully is:

1. Eating mindfully first begins with noticing if you are actually even hungry.
2. It involves asking your body what it needs to satisfy this hunger and carefully listening to its response.
3. Mindful eating is about being present and cognizant of the eating.
4. It is actually tasting what is in your mouth, noticing the colors, flavors and textures of the food.
5. It is about being aware of each bite, each chew, and the feeling of the food sliding down the throat as it is being swallowed.

6. Eating mindfully is about enjoying and savoring every bite.
7. It is about checking-in and noticing when the symptoms of hunger stop and the signs of satiation begin.
8. It is about noticing when you are no longer hungry and being present enough to stop eating when the feeling of hunger has been gratified. It is awareness that hunger is no longer present.
9. Eating mindfully is about knowing if you are really eating out of hunger, or if the eating is coming from boredom, stress, frustration, sadness, or depression.
10. It is knowing whether you are actually really thirsty rather than hungry. Is your mouth dry?
11. It is about noticing how you feel while you are eating. What is your emotional or feeling tone? Are the foods that you have chosen satisfying your hunger?
12. It is about noticing how you feel after having eaten. How did the food make you feel? Are you energized, sluggish, sleepy, heavy, and queasy? Did you get heartburn or gas? A headache?
13. It is about your brain knowing you are eating, not just your mouth.
14. It is about knowing if it is food you are craving, or is it attention, or comfort or love?
15. It is about eating intentionally for energy, health and vitality.

What mindful eating is not:

1. Eating mindfully is not forgetting to eat until you find yourself famished, shaky or weak with hunger.
2. It is not "cleaning your plate" because that's what you are "supposed to do".
3. It is not eating until you realize you are stuffed.
4. Eating mindfully is not eating in the car, at the computer, or in front of the TV.
5. Eating mindfully is not eating standing at the counter or at the kitchen sink.
6. It is not cramming down food in a hurry.

7. It's not eating things just because they taste good, without making an intelligent assessment of how they will affect your mind-body system.
8. It is not eating things you don't like just because you are on a "diet".
9. It is not eating just to be eating.
10. It is not suddenly discovering you have finished a whole pint of ice cream.

I had the experience of living in France for close to 2 years. Interestingly, as many others have, I observed that the French are not fat. The only fat people I noticed in France were the American tourists! I began to observe French friends eating and even inquired of the French people about their eating. One thing they repeatedly told me was that they never eat while in a car, or watching TV, on the computer, or while standing up at the kitchen counter! They always sit down and are present to the meal. There is a "reverence" if you will towards eating in France, and this reverence translates into a certain degree of mindfulness that is present when eating in their culture. They luxuriate over the food. The brain knows they are eating, the mouth, the eyes, the nose, the tongue, and the hands, all the senses know that food is being taken in. I believe this act of awareness and presence prevents them from mindlessly over-eating. I believe if the brain and the five senses know that eating has taken place, you are less likely to end up snacking an hour or two later.

Mindful Eating Exercise by Jesse Foy, MSOM, C.A., Dip. Ac.

Choose a time and a place for eating that promotes mindful eating. Try eating in a quiet distraction-free environment. Slow down your movements enough so that you can watch the entire process carefully without judgment.

Step 1: Take a moment to bring your attention to your breath, body, emotions, and thoughts, noticing the whole domain of your life.

Step 2: Bring your awareness to the meal as if you have never encountered it before.

Step 3: Before you begin eating, look down at your food. Take in what it looks like, how it smells, and think about where it came from. See if you can notice the urge to eat (your mouth watering, the feeling of hunger) before you take a bite.

Step 4: Put a bite into your mouth. Notice how the food feels in your mouth and what it tastes like. Before you swallow, notice the things that happen in your mouth when you put food in. Notice how you salivate. Notice the urge to swallow. Notice the sensation of chewing.

Step 5: As you swallow your food, notice what it feels like going down. How does your stomach feel now that it is one bite fuller?

Step 6: Repeat your mindful eating for each bite until your meal is finished. Try to decide when the meal is finished based on the sensations of your body (Ex. The feeling of fullness in your belly, no longer having the sensation of hunger).

Step 7: Write down any observations you may have noticed in your journal.

Mindful Eating Exercise from John Kabat-Zinn, PhD: Raisin Exercise

In his book, <u>Coming to Our Senses</u>, mindfulness guru Jon Kabat-Zinn says, "When we taste with attention, even the simplest foods provide a universe of sensory experience, awakening us to them."

"The Raisin Consciousness" is an exercise Jon Kabat-Zinn uses with his clients as an introductory exercise in mindfulness meditation experience. For many people, although they have eaten raisins many times, this meditation is perhaps the first time they have really tasted a raisin. (Note: if you don't like raisins, you can use another fruit or nut.)

Raisin Meditation

1. Sit comfortably in a chair.
2. Place a raisin in your hand.
3. Examine the raisin as if you have never seen it before.
4. Imagine it as its "plump self" growing on the vine surrounded by nature.

5. As you look at the raisin, become conscious of what you see: the shape, texture, color and size. Is it hard or soft?
6. Bring the raisin to your nose and smell it.
7. Are you anticipating eating the raisin? Is it difficult not to just pop it in your mouth?
8. How does the raisin feel? How small is it in your hand?
9. Place the raisin in your mouth. Become aware of what your tongue is doing.
10. Bite ever so lightly into the raisin. Feel its squishiness.
11. Chew three times and then stop.
12. Describe the flavor of the raisin. What is the texture?
13. As you complete chewing, swallow the raisin.
14. Sit quietly, breathing, aware of what you are sensing.

Raisins seem so ordinary, but this exercise helps us to recognize that they are truly extraordinary. It helps us to be fully present in a way that awakens the mind and senses to experiencing every aspect of eating the raisin. Was there something about a raisin that you had never quite noticed before? Completely and accurately experiencing the raisin dispels old, long-held notions about raisins, and allows us to rediscover the raisin in a new way. In doing this exercise every one of the senses was aware that you were eating the raisin. You ate this raisin with mindfulness. Eating all foods can be an awakening of the senses, special and out of the ordinary, if you are fully present to each bite and each taste. It is amazing how much tastier and more satisfying food is when you eat with conscious awareness.

Dr. Jon Kabat-Zinn describes the effect of this meditation in the following quote: *"Such an exercise delivers wakefulness immediately. In this moment, there is only tasting."*

"When walking, walk; when eating, eat." ~Zen quote

Focus for Today: Eat one meal mindfully, using the exercise above as your guide. Try Dr. Jon Kabat-Zinn's raisin meditation.

Journal: What did you observe from your mindful eating exercise?

Recipe of the Day:

Practice mindfulness by preparing and drinking this simple smoothie with presence and awareness.

Hot Chocolate Smoothie

1 Tbsp almond butter
3 Tbsp cocoa powder
1 Tbsp agave nectar or to taste
4 oz hot water

Blend ingredients together in blender for a rich hot chocolate smoothie perfect for a fall or winter morning!

Daily Food Journal

Date:_____   Intention for the day:_____   Weight:_____

Water: ☐☐☐◼◼◼◼   *X off one water for every 8 oz. of water that you drink. This includes lemon waters. During a cleanse you should have at least 3 lemon waters daily.*

YOGI PLATE ➡	¼ Protein ➡	⬅ ½ Veggies
	¼ Whole Grains ➡	

Rate your hunger, mood, energy
and after meal satisfaction

1=Low	2=Average	3=High

Time	Meal/ Snack	Food/ Beverage	Hungry?	Mood?	Energy?	Satisfied?
	Breakfast					
	Snack					
	Lunch					
	Snack					
	Dinner					
	Snack					

At the end of the day, reflect on how many servings you had of the following foods/beverages:

Vegetables (Unlimited)	
Whole Grains (Women 1 -3)	
Fruit (Aim for 2)	
Protein (Aim for 3 or more)	

Did I Avoid?	Yes	No	How Much?
Alcohol			
Soft Drinks			
White Sugar			
Artificial Sweeteners			
Processed Food			
Fast Food			

Alert! Use Meat Sparingly
Consume meat no more than 3 times a week!

List your observations and insights for the day. These include successes and behaviors that need attention:

_____
_____
_____
_____
_____

Day 33: *Hara Hachi Bu*

"Life itself is the proper binge." ~Julia Child

Hara hachi bu is a Japanese concept meaning to eat until you are 80% full. The word literally translates as "80% stomach". Similarly, in Ayurveda, it is taught that we should stop eating at 70% full. In fact, Ayurvedic eating recommendations are to fill the stomach with one third liquids, one third food, and leave the other third empty. This is said to leave space for air to fan the flames of the digestive fire. What is clear in these two philosophies, even though the percentages are slightly different, is that it is best to stop eating when we are 70-80% full. This practice is not only for weight-loss or weight maintenance purposes, but the practice also promotes better health. Quite simply put, "less is more".

In Ayurveda, over-eating even the healthiest foods is known to create *ama* or toxins. Overeating is said to diminish *agni* or "digestive fire." This fire is directly related to metabolism, and is known to be the most critical factor in health and vitality as well as immunity. Yoga and Ayurveda are both *agni* (digestive fire) builders. The digestive fire breaks down the food, releasing the nutrients for all tissues of the body. When this fire is diminished, the food isn't properly or completely broken down and *ama* or toxins result, weighting down the body and slowing down the metabolism. This fire, when functioning properly, also destroys pathogens. Studies have proven that people who eat fewer calories not only weigh less, but they actually live an average of 10 years longer! They physically age more slowly, resulting in a body and skin that looks and behaves like that of someone 10-15 years younger.

To stop eating at 70-80% full requires us to cultivate a great deal of mindfulness at meals. This requires being present to each bite, noticing the sensations arising in the body after a bite is taken. Most of us are conditioned to eat until we are 100% full. Some of us are even conditioned to eat until we are 120% full or more, going away from each meal feeling stuffed. *Hara hachi bu* is a process of reconditioning the mind as well as the mouth and stomach. By being tuned in to the sensations of fullness, we can begin to re-educate ourselves to eat differently, in order to feel better, look better and improve overall health. By being fully present to our meals, we can recondition ourselves to stop eating at 70-80% full.

During Yoga teacher trainings, we often sit on the floor in a seated pose called *sukasana* or some variation of lotus position for our meals. Interestingly, when you sit in this position, it is difficult to overeat. The abdominal muscles are being used to hold you upright with good posture which actually restricts how much the stomach can hold. This is quite different from sitting slumped in a chair where your back is supported and the abdomen is flaccid. When I return home from the trainings I am always amazed at how loose my clothing is in the waist! I have trimmed and toned the muscles, and I believe this position prevents me from overeating. Interestingly, Maya Tiwari notes in her book Ayurveda, a Life of Balance that many cultures sit to eat in variations of the lotus position directly on the floor or earth. Most notably, these cultures, Japanese, Indian, various African cultures, tend to be the slimmest. She asserts that having to lean forward to eat in this position restricts the amount of food that can be eaten. I believe that being grounded to the earth, where we grow the food, makes us feel more connected to what it is that we are eating as well. One of my students noted that numerous Americans eat seated in a recliner, dramatically expanding the abdominal area, allowing for more food to go in. This practice is detrimental to weight and health! By being mindful enough to stop eating at 70% full, we have the ability to decrease our weight while increasing our health.

Beyond cultivating awareness of 70-80% fullness, there are two additional ways we can enhance awareness of how much we are actually eating. These two practices often go overlooked. Our culture has underestimated the effects of breathing and chewing well while eating. Ayurveda finds these aspects of equal importance to what you are eating.

Many people inhale their *food* instead of their breath during a meal. According to Yoga philosophy, we eat with the mouth and breathe with the nose. Remembering to breathe while you are eating serves you well in two ways. First, taking a breath between bites slows down the eating process, decreasing the likelihood of overeating. It is known that it takes the brain 20 minutes to register the sensation of "fullness". Using the breath to slow down the intake of food helps you to make the 20 minute journey to the sensation of fullness while taking in less food. Equally as important as slowing down the speed at which you intake food is the powerful effect the breath has on the *agni* or "digestive fire." Fire needs air to burn sufficiently. The more air a fire receives, the more powerfully the fire burns. This *agni* is directly related to metabolism. It takes air to metabolize the foods you are taking in. When you forget to breathe, the metabolism slows down. When breathing is increased, the fire of the metabolism is increased.

The same individuals who have the tendency to inhale their food also tend to under-chew the food they are eating. According to Ayurveda, you should chew long enough to liquefy foods. The mouth is the first player in the digestive process. It is the teeth and the saliva which break food down in order for the nutrients to be released from the food and into your body. The saliva contains digestive enzymes, which begin to properly break down the food while it is still in your mouth. By chewing solid foods into a liquid or *chyme*, the Ayurvedic name for food liquefied in the mouth, the food is then sufficiently broken down for the optimal absorption of its nutrient contents into the body. Different nutrients are absorbed at various stages of the digestive process. By inhaling food without completely chewing each bite, the eater is not absorbing all the life-force that the food has to offer. You are getting all the calories, without all the benefits. It is recommended that each bite is chewed 20-30 times before swallowing in order to maximize digestion. This also acts to slow down the eating process, making it a more mindful experience.

In order to make sure you are breathing while you eat and chewing your food completely, it is important that you do not wait until you are "starving" to eat. Of equal importance is making sure you are not eating on the run or eating in a hurry. Giving yourself time to eat should be made a priority. The French and Italians never rush through a meal. They savor and enjoy every bite. Make eating a practice like Yoga or meditation, where you come to the meal with ease and awareness. Eat with a reverence and respect for the food you have been so blessed to receive, for there are many who have not been so fortunate. Eating and digestion were not biologically designed to be done in a hurry. Reaching your optimal weight and receiving the optimal energy the food can transmit is dependent on you making sufficient time to eat, rather than rushing through the entire experience.

Eating until 80% full, chewing your food completely, and breathing in air instead of inhaling food each will effect a profound change in your eating and in your weight, energy, health and vitality. All of these boil down to a single thing . . . *awareness*. Cultivate awareness of these three things and you have moved closer to Enlightened Eating!

"Awareness is the greatest agent for change" ~Eckhart Tolle

Focus for Today: Stop eating when you feel 70-80% full at each of your three meals today. This is easier said than done, and will require you to bring a great deal of awareness to your meals. Try eating your meal sitting on the floor like the Japanese or a yogi. Notice if you naturally eat less. Are you breathing while you eat, or are you inhaling your food? Make it a practice to breathe between each bite, revving up the metabolism while slowing down the intake of food. Are you chewing your food into liquid, or are you swallowing the food before it has been properly broken down? Aim for 20-30 chews for each bite of solid food.

Journal: How did employing this new way of eating go today? What if any difficulties arose? Observe yourself with compassion. How did you feel after you stopped eating at 70-80% fullness? How did it feel to breathe between each bite? Did you notice any changes in your digestion? Was it difficult to chew 20-30 times for each bite?

Recipe of the Day:

This is one of my favorite sandwiches, and was invented by my husband! Try chewing this into liquid as your practice today!

Open-Faced Tomato Goat Cheese Sandwich

Fresh French bread (whole grain optional)
Thinly sliced tomato
Baby salad greens
Spreadable goat cheese such as *Montchevre*
Garlic salt
Pepper
Olive oil
Red wine vinegar

Slice French bread lengthwise. Hollow out center by removing excess bread from crust. Brush hollow bread "boat" with olive oil and place under broiler until browned. Toss salad greens with vinegar, olive oil, garlic salt and pepper. Spread goat cheese onto warm broiled French bread. Fill hollow area with salad green mixture, and top with tomato slices. Enjoy!

Daily Food Journal

Date:_____ Intention for the day:_____ Weight:_____

Water: ☐☐☐☐☐☐☐☐☐ *X off one water for every 8 oz. of water that you drink. This includes lemon waters. During a cleanse you should have at least 3 lemon waters daily.*

YOGI PLATE ➡
- ¼ Protein
- ½ Veggies
- ¼ Whole Grains

Rate your hunger, mood, energy
and after meal satisfaction
1=Low   2=Average   3=High

Time	Meal/ Snack	Food/ Beverage	Hungry?	Mood?	Energy?	Satisfied?
	Breakfast					
	Snack					
	Lunch					
	Snack					
	Dinner					
	Snack					

At the end of the day, reflect on how many
servings you had of the following foods/beverages:

Vegetables (Unlimited)	
Whole Grains (Women 1 -3)	
Fruit (Aim for 2)	
Protein (Aim for 3 or more)	

Did I Avoid?	Yes	No	How Much?
Alcohol			
Soft Drinks			
White Sugar			
Artificial Sweeteners			
Processed Food			
Fast Food			

Alert! Use Meat Sparingly
Consume meat no more than 3 times a week!

List your observations and insights for the day. These include successes and behaviors that need attention:
_____
_____
_____
_____
_____

Phase 3: Eating and the Spirit

The final week of the 40 Days is all about the spirit. The spiritual side of the journey leads us closer to enlightenment when it comes to eating. It is only when the body and mind are in balance and alignment that the spirit is able to flourish. This week I am going to challenge you to eliminate all meat and alcohol. These two things are said to dull the mind-body-spirit connection. Observe this week if you notice more clarity in the mind and in the spirit, after 33 days of eating clean, and especially as we eliminate these two *tamasic* foods. Be sure to note your observations in your journal.

Day 34: Alignment

"Health is a state of complete harmony of the body, mind and spirit. When one is free from physical disabilities and mental distractions, the gates of the soul open." ~B.K.S. Iyengar

Alignment is an important part of Yoga and an important part of life. It is proper alignment in Yoga postures that prevents injury. It is also proper alignment that allows you to get deeper into the poses. Proper alignment is what enables yogis to get into even the seemingly impossible postures and positions. Alignment is also important in eating and food. Eating natural foods that nourish the body and mind is eating in alignment with how we were designed to eat. This alignment paves the way for the mind, body and spirit to align with each other. The ultimate goal of Yoga and Ayurveda is aligning the mind, body and spirit with nature, the divine and with the highest self in order to reach the highest level of existence. This creates the picture of optimal health, beauty, energy and vitality. Since human beings themselves are part of nature, it is logical that we were designed to live in harmony and alignment with nature. Being in alignment with natural laws and principles is a part of the divine plan. Nature is creation, and we are a part of creation. When we are aligned with the divine plan, everything aligns! When we live outside of the divine plan, we live in confusion, shadow and darkness. The radiance of our soul is unable to shine through.

Alignment with the "master plan" through our own unique, divinely-inspired "blueprint" ensures alignment with optimal energy, weight, health and vitality. By eating the foods we are designed to eat, the physical body or "food sheath" is brought into optimal alignment with nature, life-force energy and a natural state of health. When we eat living foods, our own life-force is increased and we feel fully alive ourselves. It is the life-giving foods that impart health and radiance to the body.

It is essential for the body to feel healthy, vibrant and energetic before the mind can thrive. When the body thrives, it is then possible for the mind to thrive. When the mind thrives, it is stable, clear, and balanced. A stable mind and healthy body are the fertile soil necessary for the spirit to bloom. The fruit of a mind, body and spirit that are in alignment is harmony. Like an orchestra in which each instrument is perfectly tuned, the "music" of the mind, body and spirit is magnificent when in harmony. It is the alignment of these three that fulfills the ultimate purpose of our existence, which is for our spirit to grow, blossom and shine. The shining of the spirit generates a radiance that emanates from within but emits visible luminosity throughout the entire being.

People who have achieved alignment between the mind, body and spirit have a luminous essence about them. When their spirit shines, they have a certain "glow". It is detectable to the discerning eye. There is just something about them. These people have come into full alignment, body, mind and spirit, as if a circuit has been completed and a light has turned on inside of them.

I once took a mindfulness meditation class. One of the students in the class was a school janitor in her mid 50s. When I first met her in class, she had an average appearance and a pleasant, quiet demeanor. Over the weeks I began to see a change in everyone in the room. But this school janitor showed the most profound change of all. During the last class, I looked at her, and saw a radiant glow. There was a discernible vibrancy about her that hadn't been there before. Things had aligned within her. Somewhere inside, a circuit had been connected. She now radiated with light and with a new beauty. It wasn't her job, or her physical appearance, or her material belongings that made her appear different. I saw her inner light shining and was deeply touched because I realized this is what enlightenment looks like. She had come into alignment, body, mind and spirit, and it shone throughout her entire being.

When your entire being is in alignment, you will begin to notice a stronger sense of intuition, creativity, heightened awareness, a sense of calm and lightness in being. You will notice a deeper and stronger divine connection which flows with ease, and without even trying. You will observe many more moments of synchronicity and coincidence.

Life will seem to fall into place with ease. Fears will lessen, and the moods and emotions will stabilize. There is a new effortlessness in living. Everything flows harmoniously. Obstacles are gone, because it is disharmony which creates obstacles.

It is essential to bring ourselves into alignment by living in harmony, rather than in opposition to nature and creation, not forgetting that we ourselves are a part of all creation. This includes eating the foods which nature provides, the only foods we were designed to eat. Nature, health and harmony stand together. When we separate ourselves from the natural current of life in any way, we become misaligned. We short circuit. When we live in alignment, body, mind and spirit, things will become clearer and the current of life will flow at its optimum in us, allowing the spirit to shine. Alignment connects the circuits in us to enliven radiance, health and life-force. This alignment allows the life-force current of *prana* to flow within us unobstructed, fully illuminating the light within. This light is our true essence, our very soul.

"The part can never be well unless the whole is well." ~Plato

"In a disordered mind, as in a disordered body, soundness of health is impossible" ~Cicero

"Happiness is when what you think, what you say and what you do are in harmony." ~Mahatma Ghandi

Focus for Today: Alignment. Begin to work towards aligning what you eat with the way nature intended. This alignment is the foundation that begins to allow the mind, body and spirit to align. When the mind, body and spirit align, you will light up from within. You will walk through life with a peace and harmony rarely realized. You will possess a new beauty and light that others can't quite put their finger on, but it will be there. It all begins with the fertile soil you have created in your body through right eating, so that the mind can grow and the spirit can blossom forth! Commit to a meat and alcohol-free week as we delve into the deepest part of our journey towards Enlightened Eating!

Journal: Have you noticed any changes spiritually in the journey so far? Some changes may be subtle; some may not . . . Note any changes here.

Recipes of the Day: These three recipes align together perfectly!

Veggie Tacos #2

(Makes 8 corn tortilla tacos, serves 4)
1 small caulifower, chopped
1 yellow onion, chopped
½ red bell pepper, chopped
3-4 cloves of garlic, minced
4 cups spinach, stems removed
2-3 Tbsp olive oil
Sea salt and pepper to taste
1 tsp Taco seasoning
8 corn tortillas (preservative-free, organic if possible)

Saute the chopped veggies in the olive oil and season with salt, pepper and taco seasoning. Serve inside warm corn tortillas.

Guacamole

(Serves 4)

1 avocado
2 circular slices of onion, finely diced
2 circular slices of tomato, finely diced
1 small garlic clove, minced
¼ fresh lime
Salt and pepper to taste

Mash peeled avocado with fork. Mix in the onions, tomato, and garlic. Squeeze in the juice of the lime, salt and pepper to taste. Place avocado pit in the center of the mixture. It keeps the guacamole from turning brown right away!

Pico do Gallo

(Serves 4)

2 large tomatoes, diced
½ onion, diced or 4 green onions, diced
1 small garlic clove, minced

Chopped fresh cilantro to taste
1/2 fresh lime, juiced
Salt and pepper to taste

Mix above ingredients and serve with tacos.

Daily Food Journal

Date:_____   Intention for the day:_____   Weight:_____

Water: ⬜⬜⬜⬛⬛⬛⬜⬛   *X off one water for every 8 oz. of water that you drink. This includes lemon waters. During a cleanse you should have at least 3 lemon waters daily.*

YOGI PLATE ➡

¼ Protein

½ Veggies

¼ Whole Grains

Rate your hunger, mood, energy
and after meal satisfaction

1=Low	2=Average	3=High

Time	Meal/Snack	Food/Beverage	Hungry?	Mood?	Energy?	Satisfied?
	Breakfast					
	Snack					
	Lunch					
	Snack					
	Dinner					
	Snack					

At the end of the day, reflect on how many servings you had of the following foods/beverages:

Vegetables (Unlimited)	
Whole Grains (Women 1 -3)	
Fruit (Aim for 2)	
Protein (Aim for 3 or more)	

Did I Avoid?	Yes	No	How Much?
Alcohol			
Soft Drinks			
White Sugar			
Artificial Sweeteners			
Processed Food			
Fast Food			

Alert! Use Meat Sparingly
Consume meat no more than 3 times a week!

List your observations and insights for the day. These include successes and behaviors that need attention:

_____
_____
_____
_____
_____

Day 35: Spiritual Nutrition

"The body itself is to reveal the light that's blazing inside your presence."
~Rumi

It occurs to me that in Christianity, Judaism, and Islam, "original sin", the first sin committed by humankind, involved food! In the Garden of Eden, a serpent tempted Adam and Eve to eat a fruit from a tree in the center of the garden from which God had forbidden them to eat. When they ate this tempting fruit, they were punished and exiled from the Garden of Eden, a paradise filled with all the natural foods God had created. Because they ate the forbidden food, God told Adam and Eve, they would now have to suffer in their earthly life, and they would no longer live infinitely in harmony in mind, body or spirit, but would face poor health, suffering, remoteness from God, and eventually death. By eating tempting foods in the modern age, we too have distanced ourselves from God and the divine plan for spiritual growth, optimum health and longevity.

A similar story is told in Greek mythology, in which Persephone is given a pomegranate by Hades, god of the underworld. When she eats it, she becomes eternally enslaved to the underworld. When we eat wrong foods, we are enslaving our own mind, body and spirit to the consequences of a poor diet: low energy, premature aging, weight gain, and ill health. These stories both exemplify that foods can be tempting, yet tempting foods can also have dire consequences! In the "ideal" world, everything we need to live a healthful life was already divinely provided in nature. Modern society eats "forbidden" foods on a regular basis, foods not designed by God, but created in the laboratories of the food industry with profit, not health and harmony, as their intent. Surely these foods are tempting, but this "forbidden" food has been detrimental to our well-being, health and longevity, just as it was for Adam and Eve and Persephone. In fact in many cases, "forbidden" foods are the cause of human suffering and death. For example, heart disease, stroke, diabetes, and some forms of cancer, which are the leading causes of disease and death in modern society, are in most cases the result of a diet of "forbidden foods." Perhaps we have something to learn from Persephone, Adam and Eve. I have to wonder if this analogy is just a coincidence.

Yogis have long been known to intentionally eat foods which increase clarity, lightness and spiritual awareness. Their diets have been primarily composed of *sattvic* foods or pure foods which impart harmony, peace, contentment, intelligence, higher awareness, deeper consciousness, mental stability and virtue. These foods are said to promote spiritual development and the awakening of the soul. *Sattvic* foods are known to profoundly improve meditation and *samadhi* the highest state of spiritual consciousness. These foods include fresh fruits, vegetables, whole grains, legumes, *ghee* and other pure dairy. Yogis have known for millennia that foods have a direct effect on the spirit. In Ayurveda, these foods are known to promote optimal health and well-being.

Rajasic foods, or foods which contain the quality of agitation, change, and motion, are known to cause restlessness and agitation mentally and physically, rather than health and harmony. These foods scatter the energy and scatter the mind. They are known to incite the ego, self-seeking ambitions, unquenchable desire and aggressive tendencies. *Rajasic* foods include meats, hot or spicy foods, fried foods, alcohol and alums such as garlic and onions. These foods are not foods which promote peace, harmony, clarity and spiritual growth, but can cause distraction from the spiritual path. In fact these foods were purposely fed to warriors to promote aggression, hostility, and anger in preparation for battle! These foods are known to make meditation difficult, and cause the ego to transcend the spirit.

Tamasic foods are also to be avoided if one is seeking spiritual growth. *Tamas* is the quality of dullness, murkiness and lethargy. These foods are said to weigh down and decay the body, mind and spirit. *Tamasic* foods impart sluggishness, clouded thinking, heaviness, and ignorance. *Tamasic* foods include junk food, fast food, processed food, and stale or rotten food. *Tamasic* foods carry no life-force and deplete the mind, body and spirit of *prana*. People who regularly eat *tamasic* foods become spiritually lifeless and apathetic. Their spirits will become stagnant.

They often experience moral degeneration and decay. In Ayurveda, it is noted that these foods lead to dimness of spirit, degeneration of health and premature death.

Clearly, foods have long been known to carry with them qualities which not only impact health, but spiritual awareness and growth as well. When we feed our bodies a pure, *sattvic* diet, the spirit becomes "*sattvic*", peaceful, clear and harmonious also. As with Adam and Eve and Persephone, is it possible that forces of darkness are tempting us by something as simple as food in order to dull and decay our connection to God or Spirit? Could it be foods which are keeping us enslaved and preventing us from becoming all that we were created to be?

It is not only our choice of foods that imparts spiritual benefits, but how we ourselves relate to the foods we eat. Many cultures around the world today and throughout history are known to bless, give thanks or pray over their food before eating it. In part, this may be due to the fact that in many parts of the world food is scarce. For many mouths, it is seen as a blessing just to have food! I think many westerners have gotten away from this practice, because food is so abundant in our part of the world that we take the food we eat for granted. Ironically, it is abundance of food which is responsible for the current state of health in our country!

Believe it or not, when food is blessed or prayed over, incredible energy is imparted into the food. There is a Japanese study by Dr. Masaru Emoto in which several samples of water from the same river in Japan were first examined under a microscope, and photos were taken of the water's crystalline structure. The water was then prayed over by people and blessed by monks. The water was then photographed again in its crystalline form, and the changes were remarkable! The structure went from looking like a random splat to that of a beautiful geometrically shaped snowflake! Most fresh foods are 70% water!

Dr. Emoto went on to explore these effects on food as well. In one case he studied rice. In this experiment he took two containers of cooked rice, and taped the words "Thank you" on one sample, and the words "You fool" on the second sample. He placed the closed rice containers in a school and asked the school children to say the words taped on the containers of rice as they passed by each day, for 30 days. After a 30 day period, the container of rice with "Thank you" taped on it remained unchanged. The second container with "You fool" printed on it was moldy and rotten.

Clearly, thoughts, words and prayers have powerful, even miraculous effects on the things we eat and drink. Thoughts and words are energy, and the quality of this energy is imparted to the things which we focus it on, including the foods we eat. By ingesting these foods, this same energy imparted to the food, positive or negative, is transferred into our own bodies. In beginning a meal by giving thanks, saying a blessing, thinking or saying something positive to the food, we affect it energetically and at a molecular level. This is what the body receives on an energetic level when we eat it. With this being said, what kind of energy is being imparted into food created in factories or in the kitchens of fast food restaurants?

If foods can impact our health and words can impact foods, how is it that we have been in the dark about this for so long? It is here and now that we awaken . . . Start today imparting positivity into the foods you eat, and don't let "temptation" of "forbidden" foods wreck your health, energy, weight and youthful vitality.

Focus for Today: Move towards a more *sattvic* diet in order to nourish your spirit. Before you begin eating, bless, give thanks, pray, or simply say positive words over your food, imparting positive energy into what you eat. Find a renewed gratitude for the abundance of food you have. Continue this practice for the remainder of the 40 Days. Hopefully, this will become a new part of your eating process. Remember that it is when you prevail over temptation that transformation happens. Don't give in to tempting foods which can derail your health and harmony.

Journal: Ponder whether it is possible that modern day "tempting foods" are holding you back from a deeper spiritual connection. Use your journal to write the words you would like to use to impart positive energy into your food. Make sure these words are meaningful to you. You can use this as a guide for all of your meals throughout and after the 40 days. Which unhealthy foods are your biggest temptations? How can you avoid these foods?

Recipe of the Day: Enjoy this pomegranate salad and think of Persephone. Pomegranate is actually a superfood, and is not forbidden in enlightened eating!

Salad of Organic Baby Greens, Pomegranate, and Goat Cheese

Baby salad greens
Toasted walnuts
Fresh pomegranate seeds
Red onion
Goat cheese

The dressing: (serves 4-5)

½ cup olive oil
½ cup lemon juice
3-4 cloves fresh garlic
Piece of peeled ginger (the size of the tip of the thumb)
Sea salt to taste
Pepper to taste

Blend the above ingredients in blender. Drizzle over salad.

Daily Food Journal

Date:_____   Intention for the day:_____   Weight:_____

Water: ☐☐☐◼◼◼◼◼   *X off one water for every 8 oz. of water that you drink. This includes lemon waters. During a cleanse you should have at least 3 lemon waters daily.*

YOGI PLATE ➡️   ¼ Protein ➡️ ◯ ⬅️ ½ Veggies   ¼ Whole Grains ➡️

| Rate your hunger, mood, energy |
| and after meal satisfaction |
| 1=Low   2=Average   3=High |

Time	Meal/Snack	Food/Beverage	Hungry?	Mood?	Energy?	Satisfied?
	Breakfast					
	Snack					
	Lunch					
	Snack					
	Dinner					
	Snack					

At the end of the day, reflect on how many servings you had of the following foods/beverages:

Vegetables (Unlimited)	
Whole Grains (Women 1 -3)	
Fruit (Aim for 2)	
Protein (Aim for 3 or more)	

Did I Avoid?	Yes	No	How Much?
Alcohol			
Soft Drinks			
White Sugar			
Artificial Sweeteners			
Processed Food			
Fast Food			

Alert! Use Meat Sparingly
Consume meat no more than 3 times a week!

List your observations and insights for the day. These include successes and behaviors that need attention:

_____
_____
_____
_____
_____

Day 36: Eating with Love

"Cooking done with care is an act of Love." ~Craig Claiborne

"The most indispensible ingredient of good home cooking: Love for those you are cooking for." ~Sophia Lauren

I remember the lunch ladies in middle school slopping the food on the trays with a *splat!* The food looked awful, tasted awful, and was almost inedible. I imagine it was about as good for us as it tasted. You could see it, and you could taste it; clearly this food wasn't cooked with love. This is when I began to make my own lunch. I remember my brother and me in the kitchen at night, playfully creating outlandish combinations of things for our sandwiches. Pickles, potato chips, mustard, cheese . . . nothing was off limits. We took pleasure and delight with our creations. The next day no matter how crazy the combinations, we took the same pleasure in eating them. Somehow the joy and love of creating together became infused in our food.

I also remember going to play at the home of my childhood friend, Linda. Linda's grandmother lived with the family, and you could always find a jar of her freshly made oatmeal-chocolate chip cookies. These were the most incredible tasting cookies in the world! Every neighborhood kid who entered their home would head right to the cookie jar to eat some of "Grammy's cookies"! These cookies were clearly made with love; you could see it and you could taste it.

Today, most of the food westerners eat is not homemade, but manufactured by machines in large factories. Foods are grown, farmed, prepared and cooked, not by human hands but by large machinery. Foods now begin on factory farms where everything is done in order to maximize profit. Cheap feed, lacking nutrients, is provided for the animals. Often factory farmed animals are kept in over-crowded, unhygienic and unhealthy conditions. Many times their life-time is spent with only artificial light exposure, rather than

UV sunlight. This affects the health of the animal and the quality of their meat or eggs. The animals are not properly nourished, and this lack of nutrients is reflected in their meat. It is not uncommon for the animals to be treated inhumanely. Cattle may be kept in a pen up to their elbows in manure. They are given massive doses of antibiotics to offset the insanitary conditions in which they are kept. They may be given hormones to bulk them up so they weigh more at slaughter. These animals are not raised with love, but only with profit in mind. At slaughter, animals become anxious and fearful. This energy of fear is said to be passed on into every cell of the animal in the form of stress hormones which are released into their bodies on the "kill floor". When we eat their meat, we are ingesting those stress hormones still present in the tissues.

I read the story of a woman who went to an Ayurvedic practitioner for help with her night terrors. (Cousens, 2005) His solution for her condition was a dietary one. She was advised to eliminate all meat from her diet. Once she eliminated the meat, after just a few days the night terrors subsided. She became convinced that meat did indeed contribute to her condition. After 9 months of eating a meatless diet, she went on vacation. On the first night of her vacation she ate a meat dish from the resort menu. That night she experienced night terrors again for the first time since meat was removed from her diet. This further convinced her that eating something that died fearful and anxious affected her own anxiety levels. This was enough to convince her to never eat meat again. Meat, especially meat from factory farms where animals are raised inhumanely, carries stress hormones such as cortisol in all the tissues. According to Ayurveda and Yoga philosophy, meat is said to carry the energy of fear and death rather than the energy of life, vitality, health and love.

In the modern age, foods are rarely grown or made with love. Large machines now plant the seeds rather than human hands. It is machines again which harvest the food. It was once long ago that farmers painstakingly weeded rows of crops by hand. Now foods are sprayed with an array of pesticides and herbicides. Produce is trucked and flown in to our supermarkets from all over the world. It is often picked before it is ready, never developing the flavors, nutrients or life-force it has the potential to. One hundred years ago, most families had their own gardens where everything they needed was planted, tended, cared for and harvested, right before it was prepared and placed on the table. These foods were cared for with reverence and love because people were dependent upon the success of these crops in order to survive. Today in the name of growing more, faster, bigger and better foods, crops are rarely cared for with the love they once were in our grandparents' and great-grandparents' day. This factor affects the vital energy present in the food.

Foods purchased in boxes, cans, cartons and trays are likely mass produced, and packaged on assembly lines by machines. Cookies bought in packages come out in perfect circles and don't even look like the ones that come from our own ovens. Crackers come out of boxes in all sorts of geometrical shapes, some even shaped like fish or teddy bears. These aren't made with human hands, and they aren't made with love. They are made with profit in mind. The bear and the fish shape are just marketing; they sell! The food industry is concerned about their profit, not about love, health or wellbeing. In the name of profit they add artificial flavors and flavor enhancers. They add preservatives to give foods long shelf life. They add bright artificial colors to attract the eye, and to attract younger, less savvy customers. All these things increase their profits, and our waist lines, but not our health, energy or vitality!

The family meal and eating as a family are important parts of eating with love. We as a culture have gotten away from the tradition of the family meal. This is a great time to set the example of "right eating" for your children. It teaches them manners. It teaches them about nutritious foods. The family meal teaches children how to chew their food well and not gulp it down. Most importantly, it is a great time to talk, reconnect and bond over a meal, providing physical and emotional nourishment. Cultures all over the planet and across the span of time have come together to eat as a family. This is a sacred time. It is a time of sharing, laughing, conversation and connecting. A meal is something that brings us together. In recent years, the family meal has fallen by the wayside as we live hectic lives rushing children from one activity to the next.

Our culture's solution to the daily race has become drive-thru, take-out, and frozen dinners eaten at each family member's convenience, often on the go, or in front of the TV. Through this something has been lost. Thirty percent of children are obese, their table manners are atrocious, and the family bond has weakened. Studies show that children who eat with their families are less likely to get depressed. These children are less likely to drink alcohol, do drugs, smoke, or have eating disorders. In her book The Surprising Power of Family Meals, psychologist Miriam Weinstein writes that the family meal "provides an anchor for the day. It emphasizes the importance of the family non-verbally. It reminds the child that the family is there and the child is a part of it." Her studies have found that children's emotional stability, reading readiness, and overall health all can be associated with the family meal. The love that is present in the food and at the table affects all aspects of a person's being.

All meals should remain peaceful and positive. The table is never a place for arguing and stress. Gentle wholesome conversation is best for digestion and health. "*A crust eaten in peace is better than a banquet taken in anxiety,*" according to Aesop. Ayurveda emphasizes that food should never be eaten while upset, angry or in stressful situations. Food eaten while arguing or when under stress sours in the stomach, and creates digestive discomfort and *ama* or toxins in the system. According to Ayurveda, food should not be eaten while listening to distressing news, watching disturbing television programs, the evening news or listing to loud or unsettling music. This is said to create imbalance in the body, mind, and senses, and harm the bodily tissues.

According to Ayurveda, we should eat while savoring and cherishing each bite. Maya Tiwari stresses in her book, A Life of Balance, that "*love and kindness are the most important ingredients in any meal.*" Without these ingredients, she says that *ojas,* the life giving nectar in the food, and the *prana* or life-force energy present in the food is greatly diminished.

Ayurveda also emphasizes that the emotional tone with which we cook and prepare food actually transfers into the food. If we are tired, impatient and grumpy, those negative emotions are transmitted into the food we are preparing just as obviously as it was in the case of the middle school lunch ladies who had little care for the food they were serving. If we cook with love, peace and gentleness, the positive energy associated with those feelings is projected into the food as well, just as perceptibly as it was in the divine oatmeal chocolate chip cookies prepared by Linda's "Grammy". It is essential that when preparing food, it is done with positivity and love. Keep in mind Dr. Masaru

Emoto's rice and how it was affected by the positive and negative feelings and emotions directly associated with it. Begin to be aware that the energy with which food is grown, raised, prepared and eaten plays a powerful role in the energy that is transmitted into your body! Make sure the foods you eat are grown, prepared and eaten with love, and you will embody that highest level of life-force too.

"Cooking is an art and patience a virtue . . . Careful shopping, fresh ingredients and an unhurried approach are nearly all you need. There is one more thing – love. Love for food and love for those you invite to your table. With a combination of these things you can be an artist – not perhaps in the representational style of a Dutch master, but rather more like Gauguin, the naïve, or Van Gogh, the impressionist. Plates or pictures of sunshine taste of happiness and love." ~Keith Floyd

Focus for Today: Today bring your awareness to whether your food was grown, tended and raised with love. Be aware of the energy your food projects, positive or negative. Are you cooking with love or impatience? Are you eating in a peaceful and loving space with true appreciation for what you are eating? Are you watching disturbing television shows or arguing at the table during meals?

Journal: What kind of energy does your food contain? Does it contain love? Having this awareness, what will you do differently when you shop, cook, prepare, and eat your meals?

Recipe of the Day: Prepare this delicious quiche with love!

Asparagus, Caramelized Onion and Swiss Cheese Quiche

(6 servings)

Crust:

1 cup spelt flour
½ cup whole wheat pastry flour
¼ cup ground flax seeds
½ stick butter or ¼ cup *ghee*
½ tsp sea salt
5 Tbsp water

Custard:

1 cup organic half & half
3 large organic eggs
Sea salt and pepper

Mix well with wire whisk.

1lb asparagus, woody part removed, chopped into 1-inch pieces
1 medium onion, sliced into circles
3 slices organic Swiss cheese
2 Tbsp extra-virgin olive oil

Prepare crust and press it into a pie pan. Puncture the bottom a few times with a fork. Bake for about 10 minutes at 400 degrees. Line the bottom of the pre-baked crust with the slices of Swiss cheese. (Placing the cheese on the bottom keeps the crust from getting soggy.) Sautee the asparagus and onions together in the olive oil until the onions appear clear and slightly caramelized. Place the onion and asparagus mixture into the crust on top of the cheese. Pour the custard over the top. Bake at 375 degrees F for 35-45 minutes, until custard is firm in center.

Daily Food Journal

Date:_____ Intention for the day:_____ Weight:_____

Water: ☐☐☐◼◼◼◼◼ *X off one water for every 8 oz. of water that you drink. This includes lemon waters. During a cleanse you should have at least 3 lemon waters daily.*

YOGI PLATE ➡

¼ Protein ➡
½ Veggies ⬅
¼ Whole Grains ➡

Rate your hunger, mood, energy
and after meal satisfaction

1=Low   2=Average   3=High

Time	Meal/ Snack	Food/ Beverage	Hungry?	Mood?	Energy?	Satisfied?
	Breakfast					
	Snack					
	Lunch					
	Snack					
	Dinner					
	Snack					

At the end of the day, reflect on how many servings you had of the following foods/beverages:

Vegetables (Unlimited)	
Whole Grains (Women 1 -3)	
Fruit (Aim for 2)	
Protein (Aim for 3 or more)	

Did I Avoid?	Yes	No	How Much?
Alcohol			
Soft Drinks			
White Sugar			
Artificial Sweeteners			
Processed Food			
Fast Food			

Alert! Use Meat Sparingly

Consume meat no more than 3 times a week!

List your observations and insights for the day. These include successes and behaviors that need attention:

_____
_____
_____
_____
_____

Day 37: Feeding the Spirit

"In minds crammed with thoughts, organs clogged with toxins, and bodies stiffened with neglect, there is no space for anything else." ~Alison Rose Levy

Imagine you are on an international flight. Several babies are crying. There is a large man beside you spilling over into your seat, and he happens to be snoring loudly. The teenage kid on the other side of you is listening to heavy metal music on his iPod, and the sounds are emanating way beyond his ear buds! The in-flight meal is almost inedible. The plane runs into turbulence, and you are being tossed around in your seat. The plane is in disrepair. One of the toilets isn't working, some of the interior panels seem to be loose, and some of the seats and tray tables are broken. Due to technical problems there is no in-flight movie! How would you feel mentally, physically, and emotionally during this trip? How would you feel when you arrived at your destination?

Not unlike air travel, your spirit is a passenger in your body while you are here on earth. Your body is mortal, but the spirit is eternal. If your body is in disrepair and you are feeding it horrible food, and your mind is distracted by noise, chaos and turbulence, it doesn't make for a very pleasant journey for your spirit. In this kind of environment, the spirit is unable to thrive; it is just hanging on for dear life. What kind of customer service are you providing your spirit on this journey?

Now imagine that you are sailing on a luxury cruise ship. The food is sensational, healthy and delicious. The accommodations are lavish. The ship is in pristine condition. The weather is pleasant as you lounge comfortably on deck enjoying a gentle breeze and a good book. Soft relaxing music is playing, and your body is bathed by the warmth of the sun. You are relaxed knowing that you have nowhere to go and nothing you have to do. You are able to bask in the luxury of just being. How different would you feel in contrast to the nightmarish flight?

It is up to you how well your spirit travels through this life. Are you providing luxury accommodations, or is your spirit hanging on for dear life? How you treat your body and mind is directly related to how you are treating your spirit. Are you treating your spirit the way it deserves to be treated?

How you feed your body is directly related to how you feed your spirit. I do not believe it is an accident that Jesus' last teaching before he was captured was through a meal, "the last supper." Here he broke bread and gave it to his disciples and directed them to take and eat it, saying "This is my body." He gave them wine and told them to "Drink, this is my blood which will be shed for you." He asked the disciples to continue on to "Do this in memory of me." The Christian faith continues to celebrate this meal as sacred. Just as it was the act of eating a "forbidden food" which constituted the first sin in the Christian tradition, it is also in eating a "sacred meal" that we are reunited and reconnected with God. During his life, Jesus performs numerous food related miracles and tells many food related parables. I believe there is a message here. I believe that we are being reminded to be conscious of what and how we are eating. Eating itself can be sacred or downright sinful! Divinely created foods are nourishing to the spirit. "Forbidden" foods are harmful not only to the mind and the body, but the spirit as well. I believe that our creator wants us to know that what and how we eat really matters.

Food and eating based rites, rituals, and fasting span the globe, across the ages and across almost every faith, creed and religion that has ever existed. In this alone, mankind clearly acknowledges that there is something sacred about eating and food.

In his book, Conscious Eating, Gabriel Cousens, MD offers a beautiful description of the spiritual qualities of food, *"Food is a Love note from God. Its letters are written by the rays of the sun. It says I love you and I shall take care of you and sustain you with the offerings of my earth. If we take time to read the love letter, by chewing carefully and feeling that they are stored in food by the sun, earth, wind, water, and even by those who have grown, harvested, and prepared the food, its assimilation takes on a whole new meaning. This is a specific way of receiving God's grace, a holy sacrament to be experienced slowly, carefully, and consciously."* Dr. Cousens goes on to compare the sacredness of the eating process to a burnt offering in that we offer the food we eat up to our "digestive fire" in order to appease our own spirit.

Just as food is transformed by our bodies as we digest it, food transforms us. The right foods can transform us into vibrant, radiant, energetic spiritual beings, whereas foods which contain no life or vibrancy can transform a beautiful, thriving, healthy being into a lifeless, healthless being with a dull, unresponsive spirit.

When eating in harmony with the spirit, I personally notice an outpouring of love for God and His creation from my mind, heart and soul. I feel less agitated by the things around me, more at peace with the way life unfolds. I notice an ease in my expression of prayer. I feel an understanding of my life's direction or *dharma*, a knowing of how to move forward. I feel unconditional love and acceptance. I feel a loving presence and feel gently and safely guided along life's path. I feel moved to pray spontaneously for specific people, events or things, even without knowing why. I notice many more moments of synchronicity and coincidence occurring in my life. I notice an increased sense of intuition and an outpouring of thought and creativity which I feel comes from a higher source. The more pure my eating becomes, the more I notice instances in which the right person, teaching, happening or event comes into my life at just the right time, and I am able to recognize it. I feel increased self-knowing and self-awareness. I have a more acute sense of clarity and insight. I am able to see the "big picture" more visibly. I feel more connected and unified with my own soul or spirit and less distracted by external pursuits. I have moments of feeling the greater connection among all beings, and a deep sense of connection to all that is. I feel a connectedness to the Divine, as if He is right in my midst. I feel an underlying feeling of joy and love for everyone and everything and notice less inclination to judge others or react to unexpected circumstances which arise. I lose fear completely. I have a realization that when you live in alignment with the Divine plan, there is nothing to fear. No harm can come. These are my own personal experiences with eating for the spirit; I can only speak for myself.

It has been known since ancient times in many major and minor world religions and spiritual practices that eating plays a powerful role in the development of the spirit. Judaism, which is also a precursor to Christianity, had very strict eating practices, rites and rituals. Scholars also believe that Jesus and his disciples followed a very clean diet, which includes fasting and eating no meat other than fish. Drinking wine excessively is reprimanded many times in the Bible. Beyond Judaism and Christianity, Buddhism, Hinduism, Jainism, Sikhism, Zoroastrianism, Mormonism and Islam all have similar observances when it comes to eating for the spirit. The tenet of non-harming is pervasive among all faiths. The eating of natural plant foods is encouraged, and the eating of most flesh foods are either discouraged or completely prohibited, as is imbibing excess alcohol. It seems to me that these similarities across time, culture and creed speak volumes about spiritual eating.

Focus for Today: Are you providing first class accommodations for your spirit's journey in your body?

Journal: How can you create better conditions in your body for your spirit to thrive? Have you noticed any spiritual changes over the 40 Days? Has your spiritual connection deepened? If so mention the details here.

Recipe of the Day:

I think you will find this open-faced flat-bread sandwich simply "divine"!

Cherry Tomato, Asparagus, Gorgonzola Flatbreads

(Serves 2)

Gorgonzola is very flavorful in small amounts, and creates a nice accent in this healthy open-faced sandwich.

2 whole-grain flatbreads
8 spears asparagus, chopped into 1" pieces
8 large cherry tomatoes, chopped into quarters
Arugula
1 clove crushed garlic
2 oz. crumbled gorgonzola cheese
1 Tbsp extra virgin olive oil
Several fresh basil leaves, chopped into thin ribbons
¼ red onion chopped
Sea salt and pepper to taste

Sautee the asparagus, onion, garlic, and basil in olive oil until tender. Salt and pepper to taste. Spread sautéed vegetables on top of flatbread. Add the cherry tomatoes and crumbled gorgonzola, and place in a 400 degree oven for 8-10 minutes, until cheese is melted and bread is crisp. Remove from oven and top with arugula. The arugula will wilt but impart a fresh peppery taste. Enjoy.

Daily Food Journal

Date:_____ Intention for the day:_____ Weight:_____

Water: ☐☐☐◼◼◼◼◼ *X off one water for every 8 oz. of water that you drink. This includes lemon waters. During a cleanse you should have at least 3 lemon waters daily.*

YOGI PLATE ➡️ ¼ Protein ➡️ / ⬅️ ½ Veggies / ¼ Whole Grains

Rate your hunger, mood, energy and after meal satisfaction

1=Low   2=Average   3=High

Time	Meal/ Snack	Food/ Beverage	Hungry?	Mood?	Energy?	Satisfied?
	Breakfast					
	Snack					
	Lunch					
	Snack					
	Dinner					
	Snack					

At the end of the day, reflect on how many servings you had of the following foods/beverages:

Vegetables (Unlimited)	
Whole Grains (Women 1 -3)	
Fruit (Aim for 2)	
Protein (Aim for 3 or more)	

Did I Avoid?	Yes	No	How Much?
Alcohol			
Soft Drinks			
White Sugar			
Artificial Sweeteners			
Processed Food			
Fast Food			

Alert! Use Meat Sparingly

Consume meat no more than 3 times a week!

List your observations and insights for the day. These include successes and behaviors that need attention:

_____
_____
_____
_____
_____

Day 38: Food as Medicine, Medicine as Food

"He who takes his medicine and neglects his diet, wastes the skills of his doctor." ~Chinese Proverb

Antibiotics no longer work on an array of illnesses. We are unable to watch television without seeing a commercial run by a law firm asking if you or a loved one have suffered some terrible unintended side-effect from one prescription drug or another. There are a host of diseases that conventional medicine just cannot cure, ranging from fibromyalgia and IBS to cancer and AIDS. As a culture we are waking up to realize that a pill is not a miracle cure. Nearly half of all Americans are unable to afford conventional health care. More and more we are realizing that there has to be a better, less-expensive and safer way to take care of our health. I believe people are slowly beginning to realize that "health care" is not always about doctors, hospitals, and pharmaceuticals. Health care is really about taking care of your own health. Taking care of our health is a lot more than regular check-ups. It boils down to how we treat our bodies on a day to day basis. What are we eating? Are we moving around or just planted in the recliner? How are our stress levels? Are we getting adequate sleep and rest? Is the way we live our life moving momentum towards health or disease?

Yoga and Ayurveda are all about living in harmony. They teach that when we work against nature, we work against ourselves. When we live in balance and harmony with the natural laws, health and vitality are the natural result. We are born with an optimal blueprint of health, weight, energy, vitality and longevity. What we do from there is up to us. If a builder takes house plans and uses the cheapest materials he can find and cuts as many corners as possible in the building process, would you want to buy that home? What are we doing to our own "temples"? Our bodies are the "houses" for our soul or spirit. We build our bodies with the foods we eat. The physical body is called the "food sheath" or *annamaya kosha* in Ayurveda. When we eat cheap processed or fast food, we are that builder cutting corners. A cheaply built house won't last, and neither will a cheaply built body. When unsuitable materials are used for a house, the house doesn't last as long as the blueprint intended. It begins to deteriorate quickly, and become dilapidated. When we do this to the body, we get the same result; it doesn't last as long as it was intended. Things begin to fail.

A main pillar of the Ayurvedic healing process is food. In Ayurveda, food *is* medicine. It is said in Ayurveda that *"With proper diet, medicine is of no need, and with improper diet, medicine is of no use."* When a patient comes in with an ailment, the Ayurvedic doctor will ask the patient to make eating and lifestyle adjustments in order to facilitate the body in healing itself and returning back to balance. Indeed, the body was designed intelligently, to heal itself. Western medicine often uses a "bazooka" approach when a B.B. would do. The body is already working to rebalance and heal itself. Somehow we've lost trust in this. When the momentum of lifestyle and diet is shifted in a direction that encourages healing and balance, the body does the rest on its own. When an extreme approach is used in attempt to heal the body, often the body is thrown out of balance in other ways. This accounts for some of the side effects that come along with prescription medication. Modern medicine often tends to treat the symptoms, without delving into the actual causes of disease, which are often less than optimal eating, stress and lifestyle choices which are not compatible with health. This is the case with Type 2 diabetes and heart disease, for example. Drug companies have developed powerful and expensive drugs aimed at doing what diet and lifestyle changes alone can do even better. Because lifestyle changes are not made in order to restore health, often further health issues and complications arise, and additional medications are necessary. Many medications benefit the drug companies more than the patient, who remains engaged in harmful eating and lifestyle patterns. It becomes a vicious cycle. Most people opt for the quick fix of popping a pill rather than making essential adjustments to their diet and lifestyle.

This is not to say that modern medicine does not have an important role too. Without antibiotics, people would die from infections. Without vaccines, epidemics would wipe out huge populations of people. Lives are saved daily by our surgeons, doctors and nurses. Modern medicine certainly has an important place. Ayurveda doesn't dispute that.

Ayurveda philosophy teaches that disease arises from excess or deficiency in some area of the diet or life. More often than not, the physical symptoms we are experiencing are merely a symptom that our lifestyle is somehow out of balance. According to Ayurveda, our bodies are not susceptible to pathogens and disease when in balance and harmony. It is when our bodies come out of balance that they are hospitable to germs and disease. Modern society has lost touch with eating the way we were designed to. Instead of eating the natural foods our bodies were intended to eat, we eat man-made, laboratory created foods which may taste good on the tongue, but which bring harm to the body. Instead of drinking fresh pure water as nature intended, we gulp down sodas, sports drinks and alcohol.

That being said, not all diseases are caused by our own lifestyle choices, but the lifestyle choices of mankind. As we continue to release toxins into the air we breathe, the water we drink, and foods we eat, we observe a corresponding rise in disorders such as autism, Alzheimer's, ADHD, MS, cancer, birth defects and other diseases. Ancient Ayurvedic wisdom teaches that when the balance between man and nature is disturbed, disease is the result. This is because the human being itself is ultimately a part of nature. This is simply cause and effect.

In western thought, disease begins when we fall ill with symptoms. In Ayurveda, the onset of disease is a consequence of the failure to eliminate imbalances *before* disease results. From an Ayurvedic perspective, health is the last thing to go, not the first! According to Ayurveda, just because you have not begun to feel sick does not mean that you are healthy! Once symptoms of disease present, illness is much more difficult to resolve or cure, and treatment is more complex. Ayurveda encourages us to change unhealthful lifestyle and eating choices before disease develops, instead of waiting until we are sick.

According to Ayurveda, there are six stages of imbalance leading up to disease. It is not until an imbalance reaches the fifth stage that signs of disease present. Stage six is the most severe and chronic level of disease. Ayurveda aims at prevention from the first stage of imbalance. Diet plays a fundamental role in maintaining a state of balance. Eating foods in their natural form keeps the body in its natural state of balance. The more processed the food becomes, and the further the food is away from its natural state, the more imbalance the food creates. Fast food and junk food then would be the most apt to create imbalance in the body, leading to disease. Over-eating any foods also creates imbalance in the body. Excessively eating any of the six tastes is said to create imbalance. Eliminating entire food groups creates imbalance. The carb-free diet which exclusively eliminates carbohydrates from the diet, for example, creates a build-up of ketones in the blood. These ketones are toxic to the body and are sent to the kidneys to process and flush out, leading to excessive urination as the body tries to bring itself into balance. Most of the weight-loss achieved on this diet is water weight. This diet is known to put undue stress on the liver, kidneys and muscles. Because it has health ramifications that come along with the loss of weight, it creates imbalance.

Ayurveda is not only interested in disease prevention, but in "life enhancement". Life enhancement is not only about being healthy, but living in an *optimal* state of health and well-being. Prescribing the right diet for each constitution is one way Ayurveda aims to maintain each individual's state of balance. We are not all the same, and foods affect people differently. A constitution-based diet helps prevent the accumulation of toxins and *dosha* imbalance which can lead to disease. Eating the right foods for one's *dosha* is aimed at keeping the unique individual in their optimal state of health and balance. This not only prevents illness, but creates conditions in the body for health, longevity and vitality to flourish. Eating well does not only prevent disease, but generates health on all levels! It is life enhancing.

The Ayurvedic principle that "food is medicine and medicine is food" can be taken to an even deeper level. Specific foods are said to prevent and even heal specific diseases. For example the juice of four stalks of celery taken first thing in the morning is said to dramatically reduce cholesterol. Large quantities of cinnamon are believed to moderate blood sugar levels. Garlic is shown to lower cholesterol and prevent heart disease and stroke. Oatmeal is said to reduce cholesterol and lower insulin resistance. Researchers are finding that green tea is effective in fighting many forms of cancer. Studies show compounds found in berries, particularly darkly pigmented berries, have powerful anti-cancer properties as well. Herbs are often prescribed in Ayurveda in order to shift momentum in the direction of health and healing. These are only a few examples of the healing power of natural foods. Man-made, processed foods do not share these healing properties. In fact, many of the manufactured foods of today shift momentum towards illness and disease. This is particularly so with foods which contain artificial chemical ingredients devoid of life and nutrients. I have heard so many people say they cannot afford organic foods, or they cannot afford to eat healthy. I find that statement to be ironic as we continue to see medical costs skyrocket! How can they afford to be unhealthy? (Please see the Appendix to find out how to save money while eating healthy!)

I would like to share a personal experience of healing through, food, Yoga and Ayurveda. In my 20s, I began to experience a severe case of irritable bowel syndrome (IBS) after a bad case of food poisoning which I got from an upscale restaurant. With the IBS, I was in terrible pain from morning to night with intestinal cramping. Anything I ate would be immediately expelled through diarrhea within 20 minutes. The doctors gave me medicine to stop the diarrhea, but it only resulted in vomiting instead. It was as if my body determined all food was the enemy and rejected everything I put in my mouth! I could not keep food in long enough to absorb it, and I became painfully thin. I was terrified that I would waste away into nothing as I grew thinner and thinner. The worst part however, was the pain. I have had two children and experienced labor and childbirth twice. IBS was like being in labor 24 hours a day. I could barely function because of the pain, and was unable to sleep as the sharp cramping kept me awake at night. I grew thinner and thinner and became emaciated. I was very sick, but the doctors were unable to help. They essentially gave up on me saying "No one ever dies from IBS." After months of weakness, pain and frustration, and with conventional medicine's inability to help, I turned to alternative medicine, specifically diet, Ayurveda, hypnosis and Yoga. I began to practice Yoga and noticed it helped tremendously with the pain and cramping, as well as released the tension and stress which accompanies illness and pain. Inspired by the results which accompanied Yoga, I began to read books on Ayurvedic healing. With determination I adhered to the recommendations for healing IBS, and for the first time I began to heal! I was astounded that something so ancient could help me when modern medicine was incapable! I felt empowered by taking charge of my own body and my own health, and within months, I completely recovered. This was the start of my journey into Yoga and Ayurveda.

Beyond food, Ayurveda also emphasizes the importance of drinking fresh, pure water. Water is known in Ayurveda for its healing properties. Ancient Ayurvedic texts make clear that water contains "immortality," is "disinfecting", and is a "balm" for the body. They maintain that water imparts "strength" and "vigor", and is a source of "happiness" and promotes "good vision". These texts claim that water has "excellent curative powers" and "destroys hundreds of types of disease." Water itself is "life enhancing". (Tirtha, 2007) Modern science is now showing these claims are true. Water has proven to be a powerful anti-inflammatory in the body. It is known to flush out toxins. Proper hydration increases energy and stamina and improves organ and skin tone. It cushions the joints and the disks. Without water, human beings can rarely survive more than a few days. Ongoing mild dehydration may be a chronic disease of our times as people are replacing the life-giving qualities of water with other depleting beverages such as sports drinks and soft drinks.

Water may be the most potent medicine in nature's arsenal. The human body, like the planet Earth, is composed of 60-70% water. Proper hydration is essential to cell health. Headaches are often caused by mild dehydration. The brain is composed of 85% water. Water and adequate hydration enhance clarity of thought, focus and concentration. Fatigue, headache, and mental "fogginess" are common symptoms of mild dehydration which often goes unrecognized. The brain becomes critically affected even if water content is reduced by 1%. Water is vital in the production of the antidepressant brain chemical serotonin, and the sleep hormone melatonin. Proper hydration is known to lower blood pressure, prevent stroke, and lower cholesterol, each of which are behind heart disease, which is the leading cause of death in the United States. Proper hydration plays a primary role in the prevention of arthritis and osteoporosis. Water is essential in the prevention of many types of cancer by diluting toxins in the system and flushing them out of the body. Water is also responsible for eye health. The cornea is composed of 78% water. Water helps the body maintain a balanced pH. When the body's pH becomes more acidic, the result is disease. Cancer, arthritis, osteoporosis and diabetes result from accumulation of acid in the system. The health benefits of water are too numerous and too essential to ignore. A multitude of modern diseases may be prevented by something as plentiful and inexpensive as water! The benefits of drinking fresh pure water have been respected for thousands of years in Ayurvedic medicine. Clearly nature's most plentiful medicine should no longer be ignored in the western world.

How we eat and drink not only plays a vital role in how we look and how we feel, but in our overall health and well being. The importance of food in healing has been downplayed in modern society as we have become more disconnected from our true nature. Once we as a culture remember our innate connection to nature and creation, we may find that we rarely need any medicine other than fresh nourishing food and pure drinking water. Food is medicine and medicine is food. This is something Ayurveda understood over 5000 years ago. We as a culture are only starting to grasp that now.

"The longer I live, the less confidence I have in drugs and the greater is my confidence in the regulation and administration of diet and regimen." ~John Redman Coxe 1800

The Evolution of Healing

"I have an earache."
2000 BC "Here eat this root."
1000 AD "That root is heathen. Here say this prayer."
1500 AD "That prayer is superstition. Here drink this potion."
1940 AD "That potion is snake oil. Here swallow this pill."
1985 AD "That pill is ineffective. Take this antibiotic."
2000 AD "That antibiotic doesn't work anymore. Here eat this root."
~Unknown

Focus for Today: Bottoms up on fresh pure water! Eating and health are directly related. Food is medicine and medicine is food! Eating the right foods is not only healing, but life enhancing! Ayurvedic texts emphasize that pure drinking water is inherently sweet in taste, and that we often mistake thirst as a craving for something sweet. Do you really need something sweet, or are you actually thirsty? Try to solve the craving with water first. The texts also stress that if your drinking water does not have a subtle sweet taste, then it is not fresh or pure and therefore will not curb the craving. If you have well water or spring water on your property, then you are blessed! If your tap water does not have a slightly sweet taste, experiment with bottled spring waters.

Journal: What are some healing and life enhancing changes you have noted since beginning the journey to Enlightened Eating?

Recipes of the Day:

Try these water enhancements to help you take the "ho-hum" out of drinking plenty of fresh water!

Refreshing Cucumber Water

Simply place 2 or 3 slices of fresh cucumber in a tall glass of cold water. The result is a refreshing twist on water.

Lemon Rosemary Water

Squeeze a small wedge of lemon and twist a sprig of rosemary and drop both into a glass of cool water as a refreshing way to enjoy water!

Citrus Thyme Water

Add a slice of orange and a sprig of thyme to your cool glass of water!

Dena's Berry Hydration "Slushy" and/or Popsicle

In a blender, mix together coconut water and frozen berries of your choice and blend until "slushy", to enjoy a refreshing hydrating drink. Freeze in popsicle molds to create Berry Hydration Pops!

Daily Food Journal

Date:_____   Intention for the day:_____   Weight:_____

Water: *X off one water for every 8 oz. of water that you drink. This includes lemon waters. During a cleanse you should have at least 3 lemon waters daily.*

YOGI PLATE ➡   ¼ Protein → ← ½ Veggies
¼ Whole Grains →

Rate your hunger, mood, energy
and after meal satisfaction

1=Low   2=Average   3=High

Time	Meal/Snack	Food/Beverage	Hungry?	Mood?	Energy?	Satisfied?
	Breakfast					
	Snack					
	Lunch					
	Snack					
	Dinner					
	Snack					

At the end of the day, reflect on how many servings you had of the following foods/beverages:

Vegetables (Unlimited)	
Whole Grains (Women 1 -3)	
Fruit (Aim for 2)	
Protein (Aim for 3 or more)	

Did I Avoid?	Yes	No	How Much?
Alcohol			
Soft Drinks			
White Sugar			
Artificial Sweeteners			
Processed Food			
Fast Food			

Alert! Use Meat Sparingly

Consume meat no more than 3 times a week!

List your observations and insights for the day. These include successes and behaviors that need attention:
_____
_____
_____
_____
_____

Day 39: Transformation

"True enlightenment is nothing but the true nature of one's own self being fully realized." ~Dalai Lama

At the beginning of the 40 Days I predicted that it would be the moments of trial and temptation in which we prevailed which would ultimately be moments of transformation. These moments create friction, as we choose to go against the grain that we have grown accustomed to. This friction creates heat, and when two sticks are rubbed together long enough, naturally sparks will fly. Fire results. Fire is the only element capable of transforming things. It takes fire to burn away old unproductive habits and patterns. Just as fire burns away clay's impurities in the kiln, changing its structure from mud to ceramic, we too were cleansed over the 40 Days. We began by cleansing the body of toxins, but as the body became clean, the clouds of the mind began to clear. As the clouds of the mind parted, like the sun, the light of the spirit began to shine through.

Just as fire transforms wood into carbon, we have also been transformed. Over time, it is that same carbon, when placed under pressure, which becomes a luminous diamond. Throughout the 40 Days, the pressure was on! We inevitably ran into challenges which caused us to face the fire. It was the summation of these moments over the 40 Days that became transformational. Like diamonds, our thinking became clearer, our minds became sharp, and our souls have begun to sparkle and glisten. That radiance began first in your skin, but now it gleams in your souls!

We talked about *tapas*, the fire of self-determination, in which we take up conscious action to create change. We talked about *tejas*, the inner fire which transforms *ojas* or "life-sap" into the *prana* energy that is our life-force. We learned about *agni*, the fire that digests all that we take in, both through the senses as well as food. It takes fire to break up deep-seated patterns. It takes fire to renew. After a forest fire, nature blossoms forth anew. So can we . . . 40 Days of fire force us to make a break with the past. It moves stagnation. It makes way for renewal.

Over the past 40 Days you have experienced a transformation in body. You may have lost weight, and seen things shift. Your clothes fit better. Your skin has a new glow. Your hair is lustrous; your nails are growing shiny, smooth, firm and strong. You feel more energetic, more vibrant, more alive! You now recognize that food is a powerful healing medicine.

You mind has also transformed. You are aware of unproductive *samskaras* or patterns. You now know how to keep eating out from being an obstacle on your path to your best self. You are aware of your constitution and how to eat to keep it in balance. You are present when you eat. You understand that each eating experience stands alone, and one eating transgression has no effect on other eating experiences. You eat with awareness and mindfulness. You know it is perfectly ok to be imperfect and to start over rather than "give up". You can consciously witness yourself both as you struggle with food and as you succeed. Your mind has new insight, greater understanding and clearer focus. You now know that self-care is vital to well-being, not a luxury. You now realize that food contains vital life-force . . . or not. You know that when you cook with love, the food you eat is infused with that same positive energy. You know that right eating is a pillar of health and well-being. You are also aware of the temptation to self-sabotage. By now you may notice a change in your overall mood and in your emotional tone. You may experience a stronger spiritual connection. It is my hope that you have become enlightened as to how powerful an effect what and how you eat has on your health, energy, weight, mood and vitality.

Changing how you eat changes your life! Eating and food play a powerful role in how we look, how we feel energetically and emotionally, as well as how we thrive on a spiritual level. Over the past 40 Days, you have had an opportunity to witness this for yourself, watching the transformation take place on the inside and on the outside along the journey.

By now your spirit is beginning to shine . . .

Focus for Today:

Today take some time to journal about changes you've noticed over the 40 Days. Observe how you have transformed. Note changes in how you look, and how you feel. Be sure to check in on your overall mood and emotional tone. Check in on your energy levels. Examine your skin, the fit of your clothing. What do you see in the mirror? Examine your nails, and hair. Note the clarity of your thoughts, your focus and concentration. Note your personal spiritual connection. Has anything changed? Have you noticed more focus spiritually? Have you observed you're more in tune with the whisperings of God and the yearnings of your spirit?

Also note your biggest struggles over the 40 Days. What have you learned that you will continue with after the 40 Days is over. What revelations have come to you during this journey?

Journal: Record your observations below, and compare them with your observations 40 days ago.

Final Observations:

My skin is:

My hair is:

My nails are:

The fit of my clothes is:

I currently wear size:

Areas of my body I'd like to see change: (Describe what you'd like to see change.)

Body fat %:

Waist measurement: (Place measuring tape right at navel.)

Upper hip: (Measure area right over the top part of the pelvis bone.)

Lower hip: (Measure the widest area of the hip, around the hip crease in which the thighs and hip meet.)

Thighs: (Measure around the mid-thigh halfway down the leg.)

Upper arms: (Measure around the halfway point between shoulder and elbow.)

Chest: (Place tape around the widest part of the chest, under arms, position right at nipples.)

Present energy level:

Recent mood and emotional tone:

Spiritual connection: (Prayer life, sense of connection to the Divine, being as specific as you can.)

Sense of focus and concentration:

Recipe of the day:

Broccoli-Cheddar-Potato Soup

(Yield 6 servings)

3-5 Tbsp organic extra virgin olive oil
3-4 cups of finely chopped organic broccoli
1 medium organic yellow onion, chopped
2 cloves garlic, chopped
3 small organic russet potatoes, peeled and chopped into ½ inch cubes
2 cups freshly shredded sharp cheddar
3 Tbsp all purpose flour
2 cups organic vegetable broth
2 cups organic 1% milk
½ tsp dry mustard
Sea salt and pepper to taste

Heat olive oil in large Dutch oven. Add onion, garlic, broccoli and potatoes, and sauté until well softened. Season with salt and pepper. Add the flour and mix well. Stir in vegetable broth and thicken. Stir in milk and thicken. Gradually add the cheese, stirring it in. Sprinkle in dry mustard and salt and pepper again to taste. Simmer 3-5 minutes more and then serve immediately.

Daily Food Journal

Date:_____   Intention for the day:_____   Weight:_____

Water: ⬜⬜⬜⬛⬛⬛⬛⬛   *X off one water for every 8 oz. of water that you drink. This includes lemon waters. During a cleanse you should have at least 3 lemon waters daily.*

YOGI PLATE	➡	¼ Protein ➡ ½ Veggies ⬅ ¼ Whole Grains ➡

Rate your hunger, mood, energy
and after meal satisfaction
1=Low   2=Average   3=High

Time	Meal/Snack	Food/Beverage	Hungry?	Mood?	Energy?	Satisfied?
	Breakfast					
	Snack					
	Lunch					
	Snack					
	Dinner					
	Snack					

At the end of the day, reflect on how many servings you had of the following foods/beverages:

Vegetables (Unlimited)	
Whole Grains (Women 1 -3)	
Fruit (Aim for 2)	
Protein (Aim for 3 or more)	

Did I Avoid?	Yes	No	How Much?
Alcohol			
Soft Drinks			
White Sugar			
Artificial Sweeteners			
Processed Food			
Fast Food			

Alert! Use Meat Sparingly
Consume meat no more than 3 times a week!

List your observations and insights for the day. These include successes and behaviors that need attention:

_____
_____
_____
_____
_____

Day 40: Enlightenment

"Enlightenment will be now the beginning, not the end; the beginning of a non-ending process in all dimensions of richness." ~Osho

Enlightenment can be described as the attainment of knowledge, insight or illumination which frees us from a state of unawareness, and opens us to a higher and more profound understanding. Over the last 40 Days we have attained new insights and understanding when it comes to eating and food as it relates to our mind, body and spirit. We began with the body and aligned our eating with nature. Then we moved to the mind and discovered how the mind affects our eating and how our eating affects our mind. Finally we moved to the spirit and became aware of how eating ultimately affects the spirit. We now realize that the body and the mind must be in harmony before the spirit can shine.

Seeds have been planted over the past 40 Days. It is now up to you whether you continue to nourish their growth in your life. It is up to you to choose whether they will thrive. Enlightenment is a state of being. Once we find the light why return to a state of darkness and inertia? Enlightenment is growth. You are like a seed that has emerged from the darkness underneath the soil, and you now know the beauty and warmth of the light. Not to blossom is to wither. Human beings truly are seeds. From conception, we are seeds planted in our mothers' wombs. Even in this form, we hold the entire blueprint of who we are to become. We are planted full of possibility and with the proper nourishment, light, water and food, we will eventually become the magnificent beings we were created to be. In our fullness we are capable of bearing an abundance of great fruit in our lives.

With this in mind, continue to expand and grow and become the fully-blossomed being you were created to be. We each need constant tending and care in order to thrive. Nourish yourself body, mind and spirit; care for yourself and continue to grow towards the light! A life of health, radiance and vitality is your reward! The fruits you will bear are your gifts to us all. Imagine a world in which each and every person is well tended, cared for and nourished; a world in which everyone is growing and thriving and bearing great fruits. This is the world in which we were meant to live, and we have begun to create this world starting with ourselves.

"Personal transformation can and does have global effects. As we go, so goes the world, for the world is us. The revolution that will save the world is ultimately a personal one." ~Marianne Williamson

Recipe of the Day: Use the "seeds" I have given you and "water" them each day. Watch them sprout and grow!

Grow Your Own Sprouts

1. Place 1 Tbsp sprout seeds into glass jar.
2. Cover top with piece of panty hose secured with rubber band.
3. Water through top and drain the water through pantyhose at top.
4. Water 1 time per day and drain excess water out.
5. After 3 to 4 days, seeds will sprout.
6. Continue to water and drain daily until sprouts reach top of jar.
7. Place in refrigerator and enjoy on salads and sandwiches.

Sprouted foods are extremely high in *prana* because the potential energy of their seed form is just being released.

Daily Food Journal

Date:_____   Intention for the day:_____   Weight:_____

Water: ⬜⬜⬜⬛⬛⬛⬛   *X off one water for every 8 oz. of water that you drink. This includes lemon waters. During a cleanse you should have at least 3 lemon waters daily.*

YOGI PLATE	⮕	¼ Protein ⮕ / ⬅ ½ Veggies / ¼ Whole Grains ⮕

Rate your hunger, mood, energy and after meal satisfaction
1=Low   2=Average   3=High

Time	Meal/Snack	Food/Beverage	Hungry?	Mood?	Energy?	Satisfied?
	Breakfast					
	Snack					
	Lunch					
	Snack					
	Dinner					
	Snack					

At the end of the day, reflect on how many servings you had of the following foods/beverages:

Vegetables (Unlimited)	
Whole Grains (Women 1 -3)	
Fruit (Aim for 2)	
Protein (Aim for 3 or more)	

Did I Avoid?	Yes	No	How Much?
Alcohol			
Soft Drinks			
White Sugar			
Artificial Sweeteners			
Processed Food			
Fast Food			

Alert! Use Meat Sparingly

Consume meat no more than 3 times a week!

List your observations and insights for the day. These include successes and behaviors that need attention:

_____
_____
_____
_____
_____

New Beginning

"You are today where your thoughts have brought you; you will be tomorrow where your thoughts take you." ~James Allen

How do you continue after the 40 Days have ended? At the beginning of the book I told you that is takes 40 days to reset the body, mind and spirit in order to form new habits and new patterns of living and being. You have established new patterns along with new ways of thinking about eating and food. You have learned much, but how do you keep from falling back into old patterns and habits? I invite you to continually "start over". If you find yourself returning to old ways, go back to the 3-day cleanse to press the "reset" button. Periodically, I recommend that you repeat the 40 Days. This has been very helpful to me, personally. Each time I repeat the 40 Days, I find that better eating choices and patterns and habits solidify a bit more. I find myself fine tuning and deepening the practice of Enlightened Eating. I find Lent a powerful time to commit to the 40 days each and every year. It deepens my Lenten experience, cleanses my body, sharpens my mind, and awakens my spirit. Enlightened Eating is a lifelong practice. As with Yoga, or anything else in life, practice makes perfect. Now is the time to set a lifelong intention to care for your body, the home for your spirit while here on this earth. It is your own personal temple created in God's own image and likeness. All we need to keep the body, mind and spirit functioning in its fullness and in its magnificence has been provided through nature. By taking care of this body, it can become the most stunning, pure, clean and breath-taking beautiful manifestation of who you are, timeless inside and out!

"What you are is what you have been, what you will be is what you do now." ~Buddha

At the end of a Yoga class, we close by honoring each other with the salutation *"namaste"* which literally means "I honor the light within you as I honor the light within me." So it is in this way that I will close the 40 Days. *Namaste . . . .*

Appendix 1:
Suggested Grocery List

There is absolutely nothing you must buy for the 40 Days, but this list gives you some ideas and a starting point as you begin to restock your shelves.

Breads: organic is preferable.
    Ezekiel bread
    Whole grain breads
    Sprouted breads

Grains: organic is preferable.
    Barley
    Black rice
    Brown rice
    Bulger wheat
    Faro
    Millet
    Organic oatmeal
    Quinoa
    Steel cut oats
    Whole wheat couscous

Legumes: preferably frozen or dried, not in can, organic when available.
    Black beans
    Black-eye peas
    Chick peas
    Edamame
    Lentils
    Mung beans-most balancing
    Peas

Dairy: organic when possible, if available.

Butter (*Ghee*, if available, is considered medicinal in Ayurveda)

Cheeses (Do not buy pre-shredded cheese. It is treated with mold-inhibitors and anti-coagulants.)

Cottage cheese

Eggs (organic, cage free)

Milk or goat's milk

Ricotta cheese

Yogurt (Greek yogurt has double the protein of regular yogurt.)

Nuts and seeds:

Almond butter

Almonds

Cashews (organic if possible)

Coconut

Macadamia nuts

Peanuts (organic if possible)

Pecans

Pine nuts

Pistachios (organic if possible)

Poppy seeds

Pumpkin seeds

Sesame seeds

Sunflower seeds

Walnuts

Oils:

Canola oil (only if expeller pressed, otherwise chemical solvents are used to extract oil from the seed)

Coconut oil

Extra-virgin olive oil

Grape seed oil

Hempseed oil

Sesame oil

Walnut oil

Condiments:
All-natural mayonnaise
Black pepper
Coconut aminos
Grated coconut
Olives
Organic mayonnaise
Rice vinager
Sea salt
Tamari
Veganaise

Sweeteners:
Agave
Maple syrup
Molasses
Raw Honey
Raw sugar
Stevia

The "Dirty Dozen" TM (provided by EWG, Environmental Working Group, Shopper's Guide to Pesticides in Produce)-fruits and vegetables you should always buy organic: (in alphabetic order)

1. Apples
2. Bell peppers
3. Blueberries
4. Celery
5. Grapes
6. Lettuce
7. Nectarines
8. Peaches
9. Pears
10. Potatoes
11. Spinach
12. Strawberries

The "Clean Fifteen" TM-(According to EWG-the Environmental Working Group Shopper's Guide to Pesticides in Produce) fruits and vegetables safe to buy non-organic:

1. Asparagus
2. Avocado
3. Cabbage
4. Cantaloupe
5. Corn
6. Eggplant
7. Grapefruit
8. Kiwi
9. Mangoes
10. Mushrooms
11. Onions
12. Pineapple
13. Sweet peas
14. Sweet potatoes
15. Watermelon

The following fruits and vegetables are preferably organic if available and affordable. These items are not the worst offenders, but have been shown to have pesticide contamination:

1. Bananas
2. Broccoli
3. Blueberries
4. Cabbage
5. Cantaloupe
6. Carrots
7. Corn
8. Cucumbers
9. Eggplant
10. Grapefruit
11. Green beans
12. Honeydew melon
13. Hot peppers
14. Lemon
15. Mushrooms
16. Oranges

17. Papaya
18. Plums
19. Sweet potatoes
20. Tangerines
21. Tomatoes
22. Watermelon
23. Winter squash

Juices:

Buy fresh citrus and juice yourself with a citrus juicer.
Organic juices
Use a Vitamix or Blendtec to create your own juice concoctions.

Meats:

Free-range grass-fed mutton
Free-range poultry
Grass-fed beef
Lunch meats (Most of these are preserved with nitrates and nitrites. Many of these are very processed. Look for those preservative free all-natural lunch meats if lunch meat is a necessity.)
Pork (The least clean of all meat-I recommend avoiding pork products over the next 40 days.)
Venison

Some great substitutions:

1. For tortillas—preservative-free whole wheat tortillas
2. For alcoholic beverages—calming teas such Kava tea, or other calming infusions.
3. For wine-pomegranate juice or grape juice mixed with purified water or sparkling mineral water.
4. For sodas—try sparkling mineral water with a squeeze of lime or lemon.
5. For white pasta—whole grain pasta.
6. For white rice or minute rice- brown, black or wild rice.

Appendix 2: Easy Guide to the 3-Day Cleanse

Begin every day with hot lemon water. Make sure you have 2 additional cups during day.

Foods to Avoid

*Junk Food

*Fast Food

*Meat

*Eggs
*Non-organic food (as possible)

*Desserts
*Fast Food

*Processed Foods

*Canned Foods

*Frozen Dinners

*Leftover Foods over 24 hours

*Soft Drinks
*Hydrogenated Fats
*High fructose corn syrup
*Candy
*Chewing Gum

*Alcohol
*Frozen dinners
*Preservatives

*Fried Foods

*White Sugar

*No Artificial Sweeteners
*Artificial colors and flavors

*White flour
*White sugar

Good Foods

*Any Fresh Organic Fruits/Veggies

*Organic Teas/Detoxifying Teas

*Spices/Herbs

*Nuts (peanuts, cashews, and pistachios should be organic)

*Organic Dark Chocolate (70% or higher)

*Coffee:(organic)

*Sweeteners: honey, agave nectar,

*Molasses, Raw Sugar

*Organic Oatmeal

*Oils (try to find organic: extra virgin olive, sesame, flaxseed, coconut, pumpkin seed, walnut, hempseed, sunflower seed, grapeseed)

*Any Whole Grains (bulgur, quinoa, black rice, whole wheat, whole oats, faro, barley, millet)

* Soups(use organic veggie stock)

*Instead of Soy: liquid aminos

*Organic dairy (yogurt, butter, cheese)

*Snacks: KIND Bars, LARA bars, Pro bars, nuts, seeds, fruit

Appendix 3: Enlightened Recipe Index

Appendix 4:
Frequently Asked Questions

1. **How long should I wait to eat or drink after ingesting the lemon water in the morning?**

    There is no need to wait longer than 10-20 minutes. Since the stomach and small intestine are empty, the lemon water absorbs into the body quickly. Once the lemon water reaches the large intestine peristalsis is usually stimulated. Once the large intestine is emptied, it is fine to eat. The lemon water is now being absorbed by the colon or large intestine. The food you are eating is first broken down in the stomach, and then in the small intestine. Which means it will take a while to reach the large intestine. It will have plenty of time to absorb there, while the food you ate is being digested.

2. **Can I substitute organic limes for lemons in the hot lemon water?**

    Limes do have some of the same detoxifying properties as lemons, but lemon is the better detoxifier particularly because it detoxifies the blood and liver better than limes. Lemons will give better results, however, I'd rather you use an "organic lime" than a "non-organic lemon"!

3. **Isn't lemon water too acidic to drink every day?**

    Lemon water is actually alkalinizing to the body.

4. **How can I get enough protein in my diet if I am eating little or no meat?**

    As for protein, I don't count grams or fret about it, but I do make a conscious effort to incorporate protein into my diet. As a vegetarian, who occasionally eats fish, I incorporate it through snacking on nuts and seeds. I love to toss beans and nuts or seeds on my salads. I make smoothies with nut butters or Greek yogurt, and I really like the marinated Tempah on a salad, in a stir fry or as a part of my meal. I also use Greek yogurt to make my salad dressings pretty often, and use cheese as a condiment and sometimes eat it as a snack. Whole grains such as oatmeal and brown rice are naturally much higher in protein than processed grains such as white rice or white flour. Quinoa is the highest. I frequently use it like rice! Just by switching from refined grains to whole grains you are substantially increasing protein. Believe it or not vegetables also contain protein. I also love omelets and frittata with organic eggs as well. Since becoming a vegetarian, I have never suffered from any protein deficiency and actually my nails are stronger and healthier than they were before I went meatless which tells me I am getting plenty of protein. In Ayurveda, the nails alone can be a powerful diagnostic tool.

I am not a big fan of Tofu, but I sometimes eat it on a salad, in a soup or stir-fry or make salad dressings with it. I have found that making a conscious effort to incorporate healthy sources of protein into your diet is sufficient. Some days I get more protein than others, but it seems to balance out. I am a very active person(vata) and as a vegetarian, I feel better than ever, rarely get sick, and feel full of energy! A lot of the studies I have read in researching this book have found that as a whole, most Americans get too much protein, which acidifies the body and makes it more hospitable to disease. The research I have read says we need much less protein than we have been led to believe! Cultures that eat less protein actually live longer!

Appendix 5: Greatest Insights Over the 40 Days

Below I would like to share with you some of the greatest insights my students have had during their 40 Days of Enlightened Eating.

1. The body wants to rid itself of toxins . . . We just have to quit putting them back in!

2. The body responds quickly to our wise choices.

3. The body seeks balance.

4. The body-mind-spirit connection cannot be severed, only ignored.

5. Food is just food, not a reward, a curse, a challenge, or a source of comfort.

6. Ayurveda is just common sense that we have somehow lost.

7. Getting skinny won't end your problems; you'll just change your focus to different problems.

8. What we want is not synonymous with what we need.

9. We are very influenced by our cultural conditioning.

10. Drinking lemon water is not like drinking acid, it is actually alkalinizing.

11. Meat is totally optional, totally unnecessary.

12. The food industry is not interested in our best interests.

13. We are responsible for our mind, body, and spirit.

14. Awareness of how my body reacts to food.

15. Awareness that eating at 3 hour intervals never leaves me hungry.

16.   Awareness of how food affects moods.

17.   I realized I am not alone.

18.   I loved learning about eastern medicinal teachings.

19.   Just because it is labeled "organic" or "healthy" doesn't mean it is right for my balanced diet.

20.   Previously, I ate too much dairy. Learning that dairy should be a condiment was life-changing.

21.   Eating with awareness is a big concept for me to add to my life.

22.   Eating for my constitution makes me feel better!

23.   I actually feel better now with the increase of fruits and veggies!

24.   That it was unnecessary to exercise to excess in order to lose weight!

25.   My joints hurt so much less now.

26.   How much what you eat affects your mood and your physical self. Just the first week brought about a better mood and improved skin and general feeling of well-being.

27.   How much bad stuff is put in and on our food. Choosing to eat fresh unprocessed food is a simple step that makes a world of difference.

28.   I don't need to eat until I feel 100% full!

29.   Healthy food tastes good. It is full of flavors and spices.

30.   I have learned to identify that what I thought was hunger was actually thirst.

31.   Eating healthy gives me more energy and better concentration.

32.   Yoga makes me feel so good!

33.   Organic wine does not have the same "toxic" effect on me that regular wine has.

34. Wine affects my sleep.

35. Bread and pasta seem to make me feel puffy and bloated.

36. No eating after 8 pm is my hugest challenge.

37. Food is your life-force. Food is energy.

38. You really are what you eat.

39. Insanity is doing the same thing over and over again and expecting different results.

40. Portion size-stop eating even if there is some food left. Take less to begin with.

41. Slow down eating rate helps with eating less.

42. Organic food actually tastes better and satisfies my hunger faster.

43. I can eat and be satisfied and still lose weight.

44. What I eat determines how I feel: less bloated, more mellow with people around me. People around me actually seem happier and friendlier.

45. Read labels, don't assume anything!

46. I found it quite easy and tasty—which made it easy to stick to. Even with a few slip ups here and there . . . but that is life.

47. The most important lesson I took away was that you CAN eat well and increase your energy, improve your look (skin, nails, eyes, hair), and shed a few pounds!

48. It is comforting to know I can "reset" with the cleanse whenever I wish to.

49. I can't believe how much better I feel!

50. I did not miss sweets as much as I thought I would! The 70% dark chocolate was a wonderful treat!

Appendix 6: 10 Ways to Save Money By Eating Healhy

It really is possible to eat healthy and save your budget at the same time! I've done it, and here's how!

1. **Grow your own vegetables!** Gardening is so rewarding and you know exactly what is on your vegetables and what is not! Having your own garden is a huge savings and there is often enough left over to freeze or can for the winter months! Gardening is also considered a form of exercise!

2. **Eat foods in season.** In season foods complement your body's changing needs as the seasons change. In the science of Ayurvda, adjusting the diet to the appropriate season keeps the body in balance. In season foods are much more affordable than buying out of season. If you are really craving a specific fruit or vegetable not in season, look for it in the frozen food section of the store. These are frozen upon harvesting and are a great less expensive option.

3. **Freeze.** Ayurveda advises that left-overs more than 24 hours old have begun to form toxins and have lost most of their nutrients. These foods are no longer healthy to the body. Many people are shocked by Ayurveda's strict 24 hour rule. They feel it is wasteful to get rid of foods only 24 hours old. I immediately freeze left-overs that I don't plan to eat within 24 hours. It is nice to have an easy meal waiting for a busy day. And these frozen homemade meals sure beat their frozen store bought counterparts in taste and in nutrients.

4. **Eat less meat.** Meat is the most expensive part of the meal, and the least necessary and healthful. Eating less will allow more room in the budget for the splurge of buying more flavorful, healthy and clean, free-range meat when you do decide to include meat in a meal. I recommend eating meat no more than three times a week. There are many ways

to incorporate healthy proteins into your meals without the unfavorable health effects that come along with meat (inflammation, high-cholesterol, cardiovascular disease, colon cancer) Even better, opt to go vegetarian and watch your grocery bill diminish substantially!

5. **Reduce dairy.** Dairy, particularly organic dairy, is very expensive. However, in Ayurveda dairy is specifically considered a tissue builder. We intuitively give babies and children large quantities of dairy to help them grow and develop. As adults we should use dairy primarily as a "condiment", unless you are looking to increase your own bodily tissues. Large amounts of dairy also tend to be phlegm and mucus forming, and cause water retention. Using less dairy allows room in the budget for clean hormone-free organic dairy and keeps our weight in check.

6. **Reduce or eliminate processed food.** Processed convenience foods (most anything in a box, bag or can) cost remarkably more, yet contain little if any nutritional value. These foods are empty calories and likely contain unnatural ingredients, such as chemical flavors, colors, additives and preservatives. I remember standing behind a woman in the grocery check-out line. I had nothing in my cart but organic produce. She had nothing in her cart but boxed convenience foods. Quantity wise it appeared we had the same amount of groceries. However, her total was over $100, and my total was $35. This was very enlightening to me! It was I who was actually saving money, not her!

7. **Shop the farmers market.** I always talk to the farmers directly and ask them if their foods are sprayed and if they use non-organic fertilizer. Many local farmers have told me they can't afford expensive sprays and fertilizers, so they grow their foods the natural way, the way grandma did. These foods are not trucked across the country or shipped from overseas. They are full of flavor, vitamins, nutrients and micro-nutrients. There is nothing like fresh picked locally grown food, and it feels great to know you are helping to support your local farmers! Another plus is that you eliminate the "middle-men" and reap that savings in your food budget!

8. **Shop the warehouse stores.** Stores like Costco and Sam's Club are starting to fill the demand for healthy organic foods. Buying these products here in larger quantities results in big savings. For smaller families it pays to shop with a like-minded friend and split up the food and the cost. I also find great values at Trader Joe's stores on organic produce.

9. **Join a CSA farm.** Community Supported Agricultural Farms are literally "cropping up" everywhere. This is a great way to support a local farmer and receive plentiful quantities of fresh organic produce on a weekly basis! This works by purchasing a yearly subscription or "share" in the farm. The resulting produce is divided evenly among subscribers and the benefit to you is fresh locally grown produce for pennies on the dollar compared to what you would find in the supermarket! I have done this for years. I share a subscription with a friend and we find that we receive a heaping week's worth of produce for two families of four for about $14 per week! That is a mere $7 per family, and this includes farm fresh organic eggs! CSA farms are a well kept health promoting, money saving secret!

10. **Save on your medical bills!** By eating healthy, you are saving healthcare costs. I have had a hand-full of my Enlightened Eating students tell me that after participating in my 40 Days to Enlightened Eating program, they are able to go off of or avert taking cholesterol, blood pressure and thyroid meds. I have a family member who participated in this plan and lowered her blood sugar levels substantially! When you are eating healthier, you will stay healthier, meaning fewer Doctor visits, illness, surgeries and medications. With health care costs skyrocketing, it pays to take care of your own health by eating health giving vital foods.

References

Albers, S. (2003). *Eating mindfully*. Oakland, Calif.: New Harbinger ; pp 21-29

Cousens, G. (2000). *Conscious eating* (2nd ed.). Berkeley, Calif.: North Atantic Books. pp. 27, 33, 166, 296

Cousens, G. (2005). *Spiritual nutrition: six foundations for spiritual life and the awakening of Kundalini*. Berkeley, Calif.: North Atlantic Books.

Emoto, M. (2004). *The hidden messages in water*. Hillsboro, Or.: Beyond Words Pub.;.

Frawley, D. (1997,1996). *Ayurveda and the mind: the healing of consciousness*. Twin Lakes, Wis.: Lotus Press.

Frawley, D. (1999). *Yoga & Ayurveda: self-healing & self-realization*. Twin Lakes, Wis.: Lotus Light ;.

Frawley, D. (2000). *Ayurvedic healing: a comprehensive guide* (2nd rev. and enl. ed.). Twin Lakes, Wisc.: Lotus Press.

Frawley, D., & Ranade, S. (2001). *Ayurveda, nature's medicine*. Twin Lakes, Wis.: Lotus.

Frawley, D., & Kozak, S. S. (2001). *Yoga for your type: an Ayurvedic approach to your Asana practice*. Twin Lakes, WI: Lotus.

Hospodar, M. K. (1999). *Heaven's banquet: vegetarian cooking for lifelong health the ayurveda way*. New York, N.Y., U.S.A.: Dutton.

Kesten, D., & Scherwitz, L. (2007). *The enlightened diet: 7 weight-loss solutions that nourish body, mind, and soul*. Berkeley: Celestial Arts.

Krishan, S. (2003). *Essential ayurveda: what it is & what it can do for you*. Novato, Calif.: New World Library.

Mitchell, S. (2006). *Tao te ching: a new English version*. New York: HarperPerennial.

OFFICE MASARU EMOTO. (n.d.). *OFFICE MASARU EMOTO.* Retrieved May 6, 2012, from http://www.masaru-emoto.net/english/e_ome_home.html, Rice Study

Parker, H. (n.d.). Princeton University—A sweet problem: Princeton researchers find that high-fructose corn syrup prompts considerably more weight gain. *Princeton University—Welcome.* Retrieved May 6, 2012, from http://www.princeton.edu/main/news/archive/S26/91/22K07/

Patanjali's Yoga sutras. (2006). Bombay: Yoga Institute.

Rosen, Dennis, M.D., (2010, January 31). More on Lack of Sleep and Weight Gain. | Psychology Today. *Psychology Today: Health, Help, Happiness + Find a Therapist.* Retrieved May 6, 2012, from http://www.psychologytoday.com/blog/sleeping-angels/201001/more-lack-sleep-and-weight-gain

Double your chances of becoming overweight by not sleeping enough based on Japanese study: Watanabe M; Kikuchi H; Tanaka T; Takahashi M. Association of short sleep duration with weight gain and obesity at 1-year follow-up: a large-scale prospective study. SLEEP 2010;33(2):161-167.:

Stiles, M. (2007). *Ayurvedic Yoga therapy.* Twin Lakes, Wis.: Lotus;.

Streeter, C., Whitfield, T., & Owen, L. (2010). Effects of Yoga versus walking on mood, anxiety, and brain GABA levels: a randomized controlled MRS study. *Journal of Alternative and Complementary Medicine, 16*(11), 1145-1152.

The List | EWG's Shopper's Guide to Pesticides | Environmental Working Group | EWG.org. (n.d.). *EWG Home | Environmental Working Group.* Retrieved May 6, 2012, from http://www.ewg.org/foodnews/list/

Tirtha, S. S. (2007). *The Ayurveda Encyclopedia Natural Secrets to Healing, Prevention, & Longevity.* (2nd ed.). Bayville: Sat Yuga Press.

Tiwari, M. (1995). *Ayurveda: a life of balance : the complete guide to ayurvedic nutrition and body types with recipes.* Rochester, Vt.: Healing Arts Press.

Weinstein, M. (2005). *The surprising power of family meals: how eating together makes us smarter, stronger, healthier, and happier.* Hanover, N.H.: Steerforth Press.

Yarema, T., Rhoda, D., Brannigan, J., & Ouellette, E. (2006). *Eat-taste-heal: an Ayurvedic guidebook and cookbook for modern living.* Kapaa, Hawaii: Five Elements Press.

Zinn, J. (2005). *Coming to our senses: healing ourselves and the world through mindfulness.* New York: Hyperion.

APA formatting by BibMe.org.

In Dedication and Appreciation

This book / material is possible because of the wisdom of my guides, teachers, numerous authors, and experts in the field of Yoga and Ayurveda as well as my students, family and friends. I have been especially and deeply influenced by my studies at the Kripalu Center for Yoga and Health, The American Institute of Vedic Studies, numerous Auyrvedic textbooks by Dr. David Frawley and Gabriel Cousens, MD, as well as each and every writer mentioned in the bibliography. I am a student for life and always thirst to know more. I am constantly reading and learning. There are so many insights and inspirations that I have expressed in this book which have come from my own journey down this path, that it would be impossible for me to acknowledge or remember where they all came from. If I have inadvertently herein articulated a concept as my own, as if from my own thoughts, when in fact they are someone else's, I express my sincere apology. I am deeply appreciative of the transmission of this wisdom, and will happily correct any misperception to honor authentic authorship. It is only my intent to help lead others to better health and a better life.

To all who have played a role in the creation of this book, I honor the light and the teacher within you which has inspired the light and the teacher within me.

Namaste,

Elise Cantrell

Acknowledgements

I would like to express my heartfelt gratitude and appreciation to Lorrie Ransome, my editor, for her sharp eye for detail and her wisdom and insight. I deeply thank friend and photographer Ella Gamba for her creative and professional book cover photography. I thank creative photo set director Katy Creek for bringing out the best. I sincerely thank Shannon Schomberg for creating and designing the Daily Food Journal. I thank Becky DeAmaco for inspiring me to add a food journal to the book. Thank you Lisa Crocker for developing the "Quick Guide to the 3-day cleanse!" I thank Marie Friedlander, my long time yoga instructor, supporter, and dear friend for bringing me down the yoga path with you!

I would also like to thank White Lotus Institute, the Kripalu Center for Yoga and Health, and the American Institute of Vedic Studies for their exceptional instruction and training programs. Your teachings have profoundly influenced my book and my own teachings, and I am forever grateful!

The book would not be possible without the insights, inspirations and enthusiasm of my students. I want to thank them from the bottom of my heart. Most of all I want to thank my precious family for their support, sacrifice and enduring the writing and publishing process. Without your love and support, I would not be sharing my passion with others! I want to thank God for writing this book through me, for the credit belongs to God alone! Thank you to the masters, gurus, teachers, scientists, philosophers and dreamers who developed and passed on the amazing sciences of Yoga and Ayurveda. What was truth then, is truth today. It is my prayer that the truth behind human health be rediscovered here in the 21st century.

In humble gratitude,

Elise Cantrell